Spots, Birthmarks and Rashes

The complete guide to caring for your child's skin

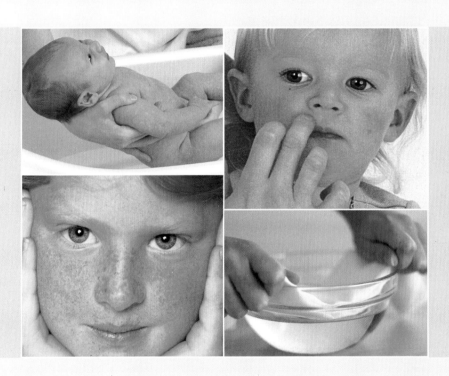

June Thompson RGN, RM, RHV

FIREFLY BOOKS

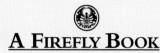

A FIREFLY BOOK

Published by Firefly Books Ltd., 2003

Created and produced by
Carroll & Brown Limited
20 Lonsdale Road, London NW6 6RD

Editor Tom Broder
Designer Juanita Grout

First Printing
National Library of Canada Cataloguing in Publication Data
Thompson, June.
Spots, birthmarks and rashes : the complete guide to caring for your child's skin / June Thompson.
Includes index.
ISBN 1-55297-681-5
1. Skin—Care and hygiene. 2. Infants—Care. 3. Child care. I. Title.
RL87.T58 2003   649'.4   C2003-901108-9

Publisher Cataloging-in-Publication Data (U.S.) (Library of Congress Standards)
Thompson, June.
Spots, birthmarks and rashes : the complete guide to caring for your child's skin / June Thompson.—1st ed.
[96] p. : col. photos. : cm.
Includes index.
Summary: An illustrated guide to the identification, treatment and possible prevention of childhood skin problems.
ISBN: 1-55297-681-5 (pbk.)
1. Skin—Care and hygiene.   I. Title.
646.726 21   RL87.T467 2003

Published in Canada in 2003 by
Firefly Books Ltd. 3680 Victoria Park Avenue Willowdale, Ontario M2H 3K1

Published in the United States in 2003 by
Firefly Books (U.S.) IncP.O. Box 1338, Ellicott Station Buffalo, New York 14205

Reproduced by Colourscan, Singapore
Printed in Barcelona by Book Print

contents

diagnosing skin problems

Spots and rashes are common, but can cause great worry to parents. If your child develops a skin problem, you will want to find out what is causing the rash, whether it is serious and how you should treat it. But many types of rash are very difficult to diagnose, even for health professionals. Some rashes look very similar. Some are only temporary and may disappear between leaving home and attending the doctor's office — often to parents' embarrassment! And sometimes a rash may become infected, making the diagnosis more difficult.

It may be useful to ask some of the following questions about your child's rash. The answers may help you, and your doctor, make a diagnosis, and give you an idea of where to turn in this book.

History of the rash

- How long has your child had the rash?
- Has it spread?
- Does it come and go?
- Has your child had the rash before?

Family history

Sometimes, skin problems run in families, especially if there is a history of hereditary allergy (such as asthma or eczema), birthmarks or psoriasis. If a rash is caused by an infection, other members of the family may have it too.

- Has anyone else in the family recently suffered from a similar rash?

If the answer is **YES**, see the section on **contagious rashes** (pp.37–54) and on **infestations** (pp.59–62).

- Is there a family history of allergies?
- Is there a family history of skin problems?

If the answer to either of these is **YES**, see the section on **allergies and irritation** (pp.22–28) and on **psoriasis** (pp.33–34).

Location of the rash

- Are there crusty yellow or white scales on your child's scalp?

If the answer is **YES**, see the entry for **cradle cap** (p.17) and **seborrheic dermatitis** (p.29).

- Are there any red itchy patches around the hair shaft?

If the answer is **YES**, see the entry for **ringworm** (p.39).

- Are there any spots in the mouth?

If the answer is **YES**, see the entries for **measles** (p.44), **scarlet fever** (p.41) and **hand, foot and mouth disease** (p.49).

- Is the rash all over your child's body or in one or two areas only?
- Does it run between the fingers?
- Is it on the palms or soles?
- Is it in the skin creases of the neck?

Travel

- Has your child or anyone else in the family traveled abroad recently?

If the answer is **YES**, you should remember to inform your doctor of this.

Itchy rashes

Many rashes may cause your child to scratch, but conditions characterized by a particularly itchy rash include: **chickenpox** (p.47), **Urticaria** (p.24), **eczema** (pp.26–28) and **scabies** (p.61).

Drugs or aggravating factors

Sometimes substances in medicines, plants or clothing, or products such as soap or detergents can provoke an allergic skin reaction or a rash.

- Has any substance such as cream or ointment been put on your child's skin?
- Has your child been taking any medicines, whether prescribed by the doctor or bought over the counter?
- Has your child been in contact with any irritants, such as plants, chemicals or bath products?
- Did the rash appear after your child ate a new food?
- Does the rash appear after your child eats certain foods, or do these make it worse?

If the answer is **YES** to any of these questions, see the section on **allergies and irritation** (pp.22–28).

The tumbler test

- Does the spot or rash blanch (turn white) if you press a glass on it?

If the answer to this is **NO**, see the entry for **meningitis and septicemia** (p.43).

Are there any other symptoms?

In addition to the rash, your child may have other symptoms.

- Is your child sick with a fever, swollen glands or a sore throat?
- Is there any itching or pain?
- Did he or she have a temperature a couple of days ago, but is now better?
- Has your child been in contact with anyone with an infectious skin disease?

If the answer is **YES** to any of these, see the section on **contagious rashes** (pp.37–54), and the entries for **mumps** and **glandular fever** and (pp.66–67).

Appearance of the spots

- What do the spots look like?
- Are they flat?
- Are they raised?
- Are they under the skin?
- Are they hard or soft?
- Is there any scaling, weeping or crusting?
- Is there any blistering?

See the guide to **understanding common skin terms** (p.6) for help recognizing the type of lesion.

UNDERSTANDING COMMON SKIN TERMS

The words used to describe the different types of skin rash or blemish your child may have can be confusing, but understanding the terms used by your doctor or other health professional will help you to understand your child's condition.

The general term used for any type of skin blemish is a lesion. These may be described as "primary" (present at the start of the disease), or "secondary" (occurring as a result of changes to the primary lesion). A blister as a result of chickenpox, for example, will crust over to form a scab (a secondary lesion).

Some of the other terms that your doctor may use to describe your child's skin condition include the following:

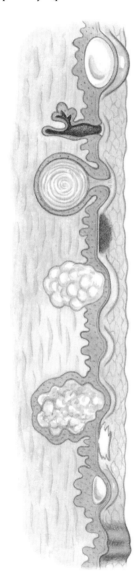

BLISTER A raised lesion containing fluid (e.g., hand, foot and mouth disease, p.49).

COMEDO (*pl.* COMEDONES) A blackhead — a blocked hair follicle (e.g., acne, see p.35).

CYST A deeply seated swelling, filled with fluid or semisolid matter (e.g., milia, p.20).

MACULE A discoloration level with the surface of the skin (e.g., fifth disease, p.46).

NODULE A raised, firm lesion over $1/2$ inch (1 cm) in diameter (e.g., boils, p.65).

PAPULE A small, solid lump less than $1/2$ inch (1 cm) in diameter (e.g., insect bite, p.56).

PUSTULE A lesion similar to a blister but filled with pus (e.g., shingles, p.48).

SCALE A shiny, flaky and loosened piece of skin (e.g., seborrheic dermatitis, p.29).

VESICLE A raised, fluid-filled blister (e.g., cold sore, p.51).

WHEAL A raised, solid, irregularly shaped, red or white-colored area (e.g., urticaria, p.24).

Caring for your child's skin

The skin is far more than a waterproof covering for the body. It plays an essential role in helping maintain your child's health and well-being, fulfilling vital functions such as regulating body heat and acting as a barrier against injury and invading microorganisms. The appearance of the skin is also a good indicator of health. If your child is generally unwell, his or her skin will usually look pale or flushed, and many childhood infections and reactions have a type of rash as part of their symptoms.

Young children and babies have thinner, more easily irritated skin than adults, and are more susceptible to skin damage. It is important that parents understand not only how to recognize and treat skin problems, but also how to look after their child's skin to help prevent problems occurring in the first place. Although the basic structure and functions of the skin are similar for everyone, there are wide variations in skin color, texture and type, and there are also some important differences between the skin of a baby, an older child and that of an adult. Understanding these differences will help you know how best to care for your child's skin.

understanding your child's skin

Your child's amazing skin

As the largest and one of the most important of the body's organs, your child's skin performs a wide range of essential functions. It forms a tight waterproof and leakproof layer that helps protect your child's internal organs, and is the body's first line of defense against the penetration of harmful substances from the environment, such as microorganisms (bacteria, viruses and fungi), allergens, chemical pollutants and ultraviolet radiation from the sun.

The skin also helps regulate the body's temperature. When your child's body gets too cold, capillaries under the skin contract. This prevents the flow of blood to the skin surface reducing heat loss. Tiny hairs on the skin surface

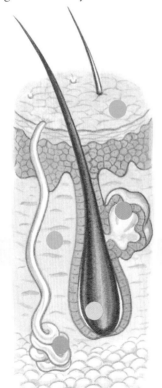

also stand up, trapping a layer of air that acts as insulation. If your child becomes too hot, the capillaries enlarge, allowing blood flow to the skin surface, increasing heat loss and turning the skin red. The sweat glands produce more perspiration, which is mainly composed of water. This evaporates off the surface of your child's skin and has a cooling effect.

Nerve endings in your child's skin respond to touch, warmth, cold and pain, and send information about the environment to his or her brain. Also, your child's skin uses sunlight to make vitamin D, which is vital for strong bones.

The skin's structure

There are two main layers that combine to form your child's skin. The epidermis forms the thin, uppermost layer of the skin, while the thicker dermis forms a deeper, inner layer. The skin also contains the "epidermal appendages" — the sweat and sebaceous glands, the hair and the nails.

The epidermis

The uppermost layer of the epidermis, called the stratum corneum, is made up of flat, dead cells containing a hard protein called keratin. These cells, known as keratinocytes, are constantly

STRUCTURE OF THE SKIN

- Epidermis
- Dermis
- Hair follicle
- Sebaceous gland
- Sweat gland

being shed and replaced, and are cemented together by a fatty film (the lipid layer) that forms a protective waterproof coating for your child's skin. The stratum corneum also protects the body against light and heat waves, bacteria and environmental pollutants.

Cells in the innermost layer of the epidermis, the basal cell layer, are continuously dividing to produce new cells, which gradually die and rise to the surface to replace those that have been shed. On average, it takes a month for a cell to complete the journey from the basal cell layer to the surface of your child's skin. This layer also contains the melanocyte cells. These produce the pigment melanin, which gives your child's skin its color and protects the skin against harmful ultraviolet rays.

The dermis

This thicker, inner layer of skin is mainly composed of collagen (a fibrous protein) and fibers containing the protein elastin. These fibers give your child's skin its firmness and elasticity. The dermis also contains many structures that play important roles in the functions of the skin:
- Tiny blood vessels called capillaries nourish your child's skin and help combat infection by bringing in white blood cells. They can also expand or contract to help control heat loss.
- Sweat glands produce sweat, which evaporates off the skin, helping cool your child's body.
- Sebaceous (oil) glands produce an oily substance called sebum, which lubricates the hair and forms a protective moisture film over your child's skin, preventing it from drying out.
- Hair follicles are the tiny pits in your child's skin that hold the hair roots (the hair shaft projects above the surface of the skin). Each follicle is attached to a sebaceous gland.
- Nerve endings enable your child to respond to sensations such as touch.

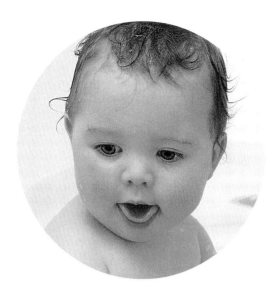

Your baby's smooth, soft and ever-so-sensitive skin gives vital protection and support. But it needs care, attention and a little bit of love to function at its best.

Body hair

After birth, there are two types of hair on your child's body: fine, downy "vellus" hair covers most of the body, except the palms of the hands and the soles of the feet; thick, pigmented "terminal" hair is found on the scalp, eyebrows and eyelashes. After puberty, terminal hair also develops in the genital areas and armpits. Your child's head hair helps protect the scalp from the sun's ultraviolet radiation, and the tiny vellus hairs on your child's body help conserve heat, trapping a layer of air to act as insulation.

The nails

Although nails look and feel very different to skin, they grow from the same epidermal cells and differ from skin only in the thickness of the keratin — a fibrous protein found in skin, hair and nails. Your child's nails help to protect the sensitive tips of the fingers and toes, and are valuable tools for prying and scratching.

looking after your child's skin

Your baby's skin

At birth, your baby may be covered with vernix caseoasa, a white, greasy substance that protects his or her skin while in the uterus. This can be washed off or allowed to disappear on its own. A newborn's skin is often greasy as a result of the mother's hormones still circulating in the bloodstream, but the skin also may be dry or peel a little, especially if the baby was overdue.

Your baby's skin is around five times thinner than that of adults, and the sweat and sebaceous (oil) glands are immature and not yet fully functioning, so his or her skin is less effective a barrier against the environment, the effects of temperature and infections. As a result, a baby's skin is prone to dryness or irritation, and most babies get blotches or rashes during the first few weeks of life, although these usually clear without treatment (see p.16 for information on common skin conditions in young babies). Birthmarks are also common, although most are temporary and will fade with time.

Bathing your baby

Your newborn baby does not need bathing every day. Bathing more than two to three times a week may dry out his or her skin. Warm water only is sufficient for the first two weeks of life. Even after this, avoid strong soaps or bubble bath and use only a mild unscented baby soap, or a soap substitute such as aqueous cream.

Young babies often dislike being immersed in water and the feeling of cold air on their skin. A sponge bath may be a good alternative to a full

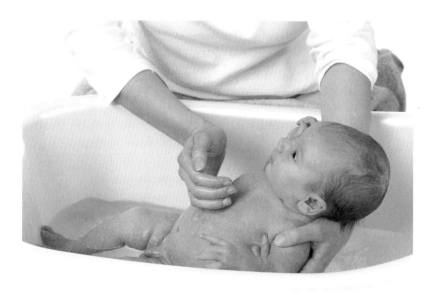

Because your baby's delicate skin is so susceptible to irritation, you should avoid using bath detergents and strong soaps.

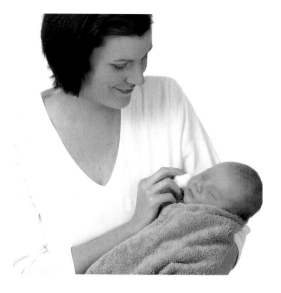

Rather than undressing your baby entirely during bath time, try keeping him or her warm and cozy in a soft, fluffy towel.

bath. Undress your baby a little at a time and use a cotton pad or a wrung-out sponge with water and a gentle baby soap or soap substitute.

If your baby's skin is dry, lightly rub in an oil such as olive oil or baby oil daily or after bathing. Other than this, lotions, powders and oils are not normally necessary for newborns. Never use products that are not specifically made for babies. If dryness continues, you may be bathing your child too often — try washing him or her less frequently to see if the dryness clears up.

Dressing your baby

Make sure your baby is dressed appropriately for the season. Young children are unable to regulate their body temperatures as effectively as older children — their skin has a greater surface area in proportion to body volume, making them vulnerable to heat loss. As a result, young children usually require more layers of clothing than adults to stay snug. Because your baby's sweat glands are still immature, it is also easy for him or her to overheat, and an undershirt and diaper may be sufficient in hot weather. Because your infant's skin is so easily irritated, you should avoid clothing your child in itchy materials such as wool. Choose natural fibers such as cotton and always wash your baby's clothes before first use, using a gentle detergent, and rinsing well.

Skin changes through childhood

The stratum corneum — the skin's outermost protective barrier — is not fully developed until your child is 4, and although the skin increases in thickness as your child grows, it does not reach maturity until puberty. Children also have fewer pigment cells than adults, making them particularly vulnerable to sunburn and the effects of environmental "insults" on the skin.

During the teenage years, hormonal changes can cause an overstimulation of the sebaceous glands making the skin oily and susceptible to skin problems, such as acne (see p.35).

HEALTH **ALERT** ...

BLACK SKIN

Black skin contains more melanin than white skin and is tougher and stronger. However it is still possible for black skin to burn. It contains more sweat glands, which help regulate temperature control, and more sebaceous glands than white skin. Despite this, black skin can still be prone to dryness, particularly in cooler climates. Changes in skin pigmentation — such as may be caused by conditions like eczema — are more noticeable on black skin. It is also particularly susceptible to the overgrowths of fibrous scar tissue called keloids (see p.26).

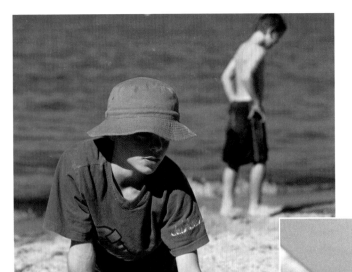

Resist the temptation to allow your child to spend all day in a swimsuit or without any clothes. A simple cotton T-shirt and wide-brimmed hat — together with a generous amount of sunscreen — will provide an essential layer of protection from the sun's rays.

Sun care

A certain amount of sunshine is important for your child as it helps make vitamin D and builds strong bones. Sunshine can also help conditions such as psoriasis and eczema. Too much sunlight, however, can be harmful. The sun emits two types of ultraviolet radiation (UVA and UVB), both of which can damage the skin. UVB are powerful shortwave rays and are potentially the most dangerous, thickening the skin and triggering production of the pigment melanin. This attempts to protect the skin by producing a tan, but even a tan may be a sign of skin damage. If the skin burns instead of tanning, the damage to the skin is even greater. UVA rays are weaker than UVB, but are longer rays which penetrate the skin and can cause premature aging. They also increase the risk of skin cancer. For advice on spotting cancerous melanomas, see p.71.

Children and the sun

Because they tend to spend more time outdoors, the average child is exposed to three times more sun than adults. Children's skin is thinner, and they may not be able to produce enough melanin to give protection from burning. The paler the skin, the less melanin is produced, and children with fair or red hair, blue eyes and freckles are particularly susceptible to burning. Skin cancer has become much more common in the last 20 to 30 years, and too much exposure while young may increase the risk of skin cancer in later life.

Sunburn

If your child's skin begins to turn red while in the sun, this is certainly a sign that his or her skin is burning. It is more likely, however, that the first evidence of sunburn will not become obvious until a few hours after exposure. Red, warm and painful skin are the most common signs. In severe cases, the skin may peel or blister, just like any other burn, and your child may develop a headache, fever or chills.

Treatment

If the sunburn is mild, give your child a tepid bath or shower, or apply cool compresses. Use calamine lotion or an "after sun" cream on the red areas, and give your child the appropriate dose of acetaminophen and plenty of cool drinks. If the sunburn is severe, or if your child is feverish, vomiting or appears ill, you should wrap him or her in a wet sheet or towel, give small amounts of fluids and take him or her to a doctor or emergency department immediately.

HEALTH **ALERT** ...

If your child becomes dehydrated, faint, confused or unable to balance properly, he or she may be suffering from heatstroke, which can cause the body temperature to rise to dangerous levels. This sometimes results from severe sunburn, but your child can also develop heatstroke from dehydration and overheating, without having been burned. Wrap your child in a wet sheet or towel to prevent further overheating, give small amounts of fluids and take your child to a doctor or emergency department immediately.

HEATSTROKE

Preventing sunburn

While outside, make the most of any shade and keep your child out of the sun when it is very hot, especially between 11 a.m. and 3 p.m., when the sun is highest and most harmful. Babies under 6 months should be kept out of direct sunlight altogether. Dress your child in baggy cotton clothes and a sun hat, and make sure that his or her shoulders and back of the neck are protected, as these are the most common areas for sunburn. Cover exposed parts of your child's skin with a sunscreen, even on cloudy or overcast days, and make sure that your child wears good-quality sunglasses with an ultraviolet filter, and not cheap novelty shades.

Sunscreen

Sunscreens are preparations containing agents that help absorb or block out the effect of the sun's ultraviolet rays. There are a range of products formulated especially for infants and children, including sprays, lotions and foams that cover the skin readily and conveniently without causing any stinging or other discomfort. Sunscreens carry a sun protection factor (SPF) rating, which appears as a number on the container. The higher the rating, the greater the protection from UVB rays. An SPF of 15, for example, allows a child to stay out 15 times longer without burning. Children should use a sunscreen with an SPF of at least 15, and preferably 30, and one which protects against both UVA and UVB. The sunscreen should be applied generously and often. Use waterproof sunblock if your child is swimming and reapply it as necessary. Even when your child is wearing sunscreen, it is best to limit the amount of time he or she is exposed to the sun.

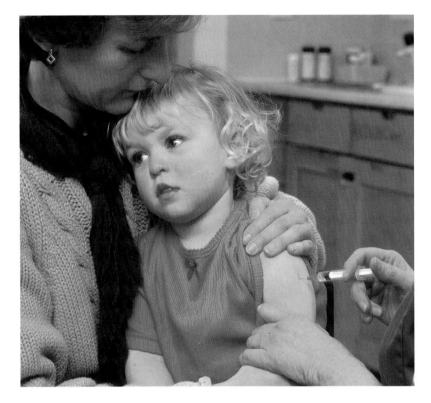

Many children — and more than a few parents — are a little nervous around needles. But immunizations offer your child very important protection against some serious infectious diseases.

Immunizations

There is no reason for your child to suffer from a disease if there is a safe and effective way to prevent it. Immunizations give your child vital protection against a number of dangerous diseases. These include some infectious conditions that cause skin rashes or swellings as part of their symptoms and are covered in this book — vaccines are available for measles, mumps, rubella and even chickenpox. Because of immunization (also called vaccination or inoculation), many of these infectious diseases are now rare. But they still exist, and outbreaks can occur even in developed countries if children are not properly protected through vaccination.

How they work

When your child is immunized, he or she is given a vaccine (usually as an injection) made up of a tiny amount of the same bacteria or virus that cause a particular disease. These vaccines are specially treated so they do not cause the disease itself, but instead stimulate your child's immune system into producing antibodies against the bacteria or virus, building up immunity to the disease and protecting against it in the future.

Vaccines go through many safety tests before they are used. Although some children do experience minor reactions, serious effects are rare. The risks from the diseases are far greater than any risk from the vaccines.

The immunization schedule

The first immunizations (called primary immunizations) are started when your child is 8 weeks old, and your child should receive most of his or her childhood immunizations before the age of 2. These will include an injection to give protection against measles, mumps and rubella (MMR), which is given as one injection, usually at 12 to 15 months. It also is recommended that children receive the varicella (chickenpox) vaccine, usually at the same time. Before starting school, your child will also need to have booster vaccinations for MMR as well as for diphtheria, tetanus and pertussis (whooping cough).

The MMR vaccine

Although there have been suggestions that there may be a link between the measles, mumps and rubella (MMR) vaccine and autism or bowel disease, extensive scientific studies from all over the world have not found any link. Since the vaccine was first used in North America 30 years ago, over 500 million doses have been given in over 90 countries, and it has an excellent safety record. Another suggestion is that the combined vaccine may overload a child's immune system. This is not the case. No country in the world

recommends giving MMR as separate vaccines, which would mean giving children six separate injections instead of two, leaving them at risk for longer, for no additional benefit. For further information on measles, mumps and rubella, see pp.44–45 and p.66.

The varicella vaccine

Although this vaccine does not seem to protect every child from chickenpox, it does prevent the disease in around 70 percent to 90 percent of children given the injection. When children do still get chickenpox, it is usually very mild. The vaccine has been licensed in the United States since 1995 and in Japan for over 20 years, but it is still not absolutely certain that the vaccine provides lifelong immunity and some parents prefer their children to contract chickenpox while they are still young and gain natural immunity in this way. It is, however, recommended by both the United States and Canadian health authorities. For further information on chickenpox, see p.47.

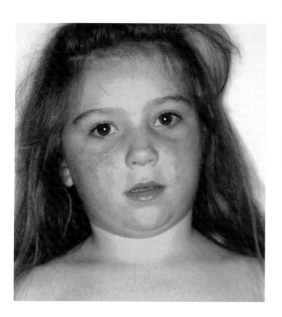

The rash on this girl's face is caused by rubella, a highly contagious viral infection. This disease is far less common today than it was in the past, a benefit of widespread immunization.

COMPLICATIONS ...

In most cases, the very worst a child can expect after receiving a vaccination is a sore arm, slight fever or, sometime later, a mild rash. Very rarely, a child may suffer an allergic reaction to a vaccine, but serious complications are extremely rare. The risks from the diseases are undoubtedly far greater than any risk from the vaccines. The doctor or health professional giving the injection will explain what to look for and how to treat any fever that may occur.

IMMUNIZATIONS

common skin conditions in young babies

Newborn babies

As soft and radiant as your newborn's skin may seem, it is also very delicate, and very few babies have completely flawless skin during their first months of life. In the first few weeks after leaving the uterus, maternal hormones continue to circulate through your newborn's system, stimulating the sebaceous (oil) glands and making your baby susceptible to conditions such as infantile acne and cradle cap. Also, because the skin's defense systems have not fully matured, your infant's sensitive skin is particularly vulnerable to the effects of temperature, microbial infection and irritants, and skin conditions such as diaper rash and miliaria are common. Most of these conditions are harmless and will usually clear as your baby grows older.

Erythema toxicum

This harmless rash affects many babies in the early days of life, usually on the second day. It is more common in full-term babies — when it does occur in preterm babies it may appear some weeks after birth. The rash may consist of tiny, firm, yellow or white-colored bumps — sometimes filled with fluid — surrounded by a ring of redness. Although the fluid may look like pus, it contains only harmless blood cells and is not a sign of infection. Sometimes the rash consists of red splotches instead of bumps. The rash may appear on your baby's face or trunk, it may come and go at different sites, or it may cover the whole body. This rash cannot be prevented and there is no treatment, but it is not infectious and disappears within a few days.

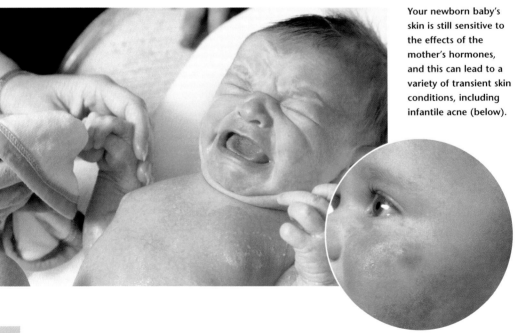

Your newborn baby's skin is still sensitive to the effects of the mother's hormones, and this can lead to a variety of transient skin conditions, including infantile acne (below).

Infantile acne

A few weeks after birth, some babies develop acne-type lesions on the face. These are thought to occur as a result of the mother's hormones, still present in the newborn's bloodstream, causing an overproduction of oily sebum, in much the same way that hormonal changes during puberty can result in teenage spots. The acne will usually clear spontaneously, but if the pimples become infected, they may need treatment from a doctor.

Sebaceous gland hyperplasia

The hormones in your newborn's body can also cause enlarged sebaceous (oil) glands, resulting in multiple, tiny, yellow-colored papules on his or her nose, cheeks and upper lip. The papules resolve within a few weeks as the effect of the the hormones diminishes.

Cradle cap

Many babies develop a buildup of greasy white or brownish yellow scales on their scalp and sometimes their forehead — a condition known as cradle cap. It can occur soon after birth, but not usually after the first 12 to 18 months of life. Cradle cap is probably caused by your newborn's sebaceous glands being overactive as a result of the hormones still circulating in his or her bloodstream. Apart from the oily, flaking scalp, your baby should be well, with no bleeding, irritation or fever. If the rash spreads beyond the scalp, or if the area is red or inflamed, the condition is called seborrheic dermatitis (see p.29) rather than cradle cap.

Treatment

Although the rash eventually will clear of its own accord, it can look unpleasant. It is not infectious, but it may spread to other areas of your child's body. Because of this, you may wish

to take steps to get rid of it. To loosen the scales, massage aqueous cream or warmed olive oil into your child's skin and leave it overnight before washing off. Gently wash your baby's head daily using a mild baby shampoo, or wet your baby's head and wash it using emulsifying cream or aqueous cream. Brush or comb the scales out, using a soft baby brush.

If frequent shampooing does not work, you may wish to try an antiseborrheic shampoo. In severe cases you should take your child to see a doctor, who may prescribe your child a mild hydrocortisone cream (see p.80).

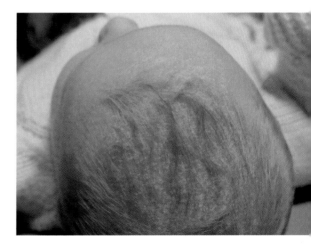

Although unsightly, the greasy, flaking skin scales of cradle cap do not itch or upset your baby, and are no reflection on your care for your child.

TREATING DIAPER RASH

1 Begin treatment as soon as any redness or irritation appears. First, clean your child's diaper area thoroughly, paying particular attention to all of the skin folds and creases. Then gently pat your baby's bottom dry.

2 Apply a diaper-rash cream to the affected area to help soothe and heal your baby's skin. Spread the cream thinly so it does not interfere with the absorbency of the diaper.

Diaper rash

Because their skin is so delicate, most babies develop a diaper rash (sometimes called diaper dermatitis) at some stage during their first year or two. It occurs when the skin around your child's buttocks and genital area reacts to irritants in urine and feces, becoming red or inflamed. In its early stages the rash appears as red patches on your baby's bottom or around the genitals, or there may be general redness. The skin may look sore and be hot to touch, and there may be spots, pimples or blisters. Usually, however, diaper rash does not involve the skin folds, and a rash that does may be a sign of candidal diaper rash (see box, p.19).

Causes of diaper rash

The most common cause of this rash is the prolonged contact between your baby's skin and urine or feces that occurs while your child is wearing a diaper. Ammonia in the urine and bacteria from the feces may burn or irritate your child's skin. Tummy upsets causing diarrhea, and changes in your child's diet such as occur when you start weaning him or her onto solid foods or

Whenever possible, leave off the diaper, so that fresh air can reach your baby's bottom and help the skin heal.

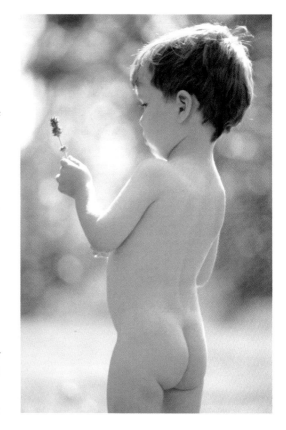

from breast milk to formula, can make your child's feces more likely to cause diaper rash. The rash may also occur as a result of irritation from chemicals in strong soap, detergent, bubble bath or baby wipes containing alcohol. Diapers and plastic pants prevent air from reaching your baby's skin, preventing the rash from healing and making the irritation worse.

Protecting against diaper rash

Although rarely serious, the rash can be distressing for both you and your baby. If left untreated it may also become infected. A few simple steps, however, can protect against diaper rash developing, or prevent it getting worse.

You should change your baby's diaper as soon as you can if it becomes wet or soiled. As a guideline you may find that newborn babies need changing 10 to 12 times a day, and older children at least 6 to 8 times. Thoroughly clean the whole diaper area, wiping from front to back and including all the little folds. Use a mild baby soap and plain water, specially formulated baby lotion or gentle baby wipes. When using soap and water, rinse off the soap and pat dry thoroughly and gently. If you are using disposable diapers, put these on loosely and snip some of the elastic

---

THE **NATURAL** APPROACH

To soothe your baby's rash, try a calendula-based barrier cream — the antiseptic properties of calendula promote healing and reduce inflammation, while its antifungal properties help protect against candidal infection. You could also try adding a few drops of tea tree, lavender or calendula oil to your baby's bath water to help calm the irritation.

HEALTH **ALERT** ...

Sometimes, the rash may become infected with a yeastlike organism called candida, commonly known as thrush. Signs of thrush include a persistent, moist, bright-red rash, with white or red pimples that tend to involve the skin folds, or a persistent rash that does not heal with ordinary creams. If your baby does develop thrush, special antifungal creams (see p.78) are available over the counter or by prescription.

CANDIDAL DIAPER RASH

around the legs to allow in air. Avoid using plastic pants as these prevent the air from circulating. If you use cotton or terry diapers, an added diaper liner will keep moisture away to help protect against rashes. Terry diapers need sterilizing by boiling, or by soaking in a diaper solution before washing. They should then be washed with a gentle detergent and rinsed well.

Treatment

If your baby does get diaper rash, apply a diaper cream after changing. This should help soothe the irritation while also acting as a barrier between your baby's skin and his or her urine and feces. You should also leave your baby's diaper off for as long and often as you can — fresh air and sunlight will help the skin dry and encourage your baby's blemished bottom to heal faster. Sit your child on a clean towel or terry diaper to avoid accidents! Ask your doctor for further advice if you are concerned.

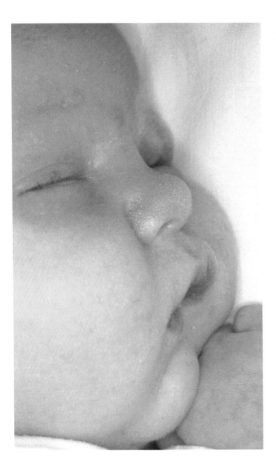

The rash can take on different forms, depending on how close to the skin surface the blockage occurs. Miliaria rubra, a deep blockage of the sweat glands, is characterized by red-colored spots and blisters, covering slightly inflamed areas of skin. Another type is called miliaria crystallina, since the rash consists of tiny, clear, fluid-filled blisters without the redness of miliaria rubra. Here, the blockage occurs closer to the surface of the skin causing less inflammation.

Although it can occur at any age, young babies are particularly susceptible to miliaria. To prevent the condition, be careful not to allow your baby to overheat and avoid overdressing him or her. Calamine lotion and frequent cool baths can help to relieve the discomfort. The rash should disappear a little time after your baby cools down, but the sweat glands may remain blocked for several weeks.

Milia

Often referred to as "milk spots," milia are tiny, white or yellow papules, caused by a blockage of your child's sebaceous glands by keratin from old skin cells, or by oily sebum. Milia are harmless and usually disappear quickly without treatment, although they can sometimes persist for up to two to three months.

Tiny milia or "milk spots" often appear on the cheeks, nose or forehead of newborn babies, but usually disappear within the first few weeks of life.

Miliaria

Also known as sweat rash or prickly heat, the numerous, tiny spots and blisters of miliaria develop when excessive or sudden sweating — usually due to a hot, moist environment — causes a blockage and inflammation of your child's sweat glands. Sweat that cannot escape causes blisters to develop under your child's skin. The rash tends to occur around areas of the skin prone to sweating, and your child may complain of hot, itchy or prickly skin.

HEALTH **ALERT** ...

Occasionally, spots or rashes on your child's skin can become infected or inflamed. In this case, your child should be taken to the doctor, who will prescribe either a course of antibiotics or an antiseptic solution or cream to be applied directly to the spots.

SEPTIC SPOTS

2 Noncontagious rashes

Many of the most troublesome and persistent childhood skin complaints are not infectious, but nonetheless can prove very distressing, for both you and your child. Allergic reactions, exposure to irritating substances, local skin infections or even an overproduction of oil or skin cells, all can cause problems for your child's delicate skin. Many of these rashes, although not contagious, may be unsightly, frustratingly itchy or persistent.

Irritating skin conditions such as eczema or acne don't usually cause your child to feel feverish or unwell, but can prove extremely difficult to eradicate — although there are now a great many treatments available to help control and relieve the symptoms. Allergic rashes such as hives or urticaria are less persistent, but may be highly irritating. Serious allergic reactions such as angioedema can obstruct your child's breathing, requiring urgent medical attention. Other skin complaints, such as cellulitis, erysipelas or Lyme disease, are caused by bacterial infection. Although these conditions are not contagious, they are serious infections and should always be treated by a doctor.

allergies & irritation

The allergic response

Hypersensitivity toward certain substances, such as pollen or chemicals, can sometimes stimulate your child's immune system into undergoing an abnormal reaction. Although the substance (known as an allergen) is not necessarily harmful, your child's immune system believes that the allergen is attacking his or her body and produces antibodies. These antibodies trigger a chain of events that leads to cells in your child's body releasing chemicals known as mediators into the surrounding body tissues. These mediators (histamine for example) produce the symptoms of allergy — the "allergic response."

This reaction does not usually occur the first time your child comes into contact with an allergen, and a substance may be tolerated for a long time before problems occur. The word "allergy" is sometimes used loosely to describe any kind of abnormal reaction, but a true allergic response must involve your child's immune system. A reaction to a certain food, for example, may be due to your child's dislike or intolerance of the food rather than the result of an actual allergy.

What to look for

The symptoms of allergy vary from child to child, and also depend on the type of allergen and the part of your child's body affected. An allergic skin reaction will often result in an urticaria-type rash (see p.24). This rash may include wheals, widespread bright-red skin, swelling, itching, or large or small blisters. Your

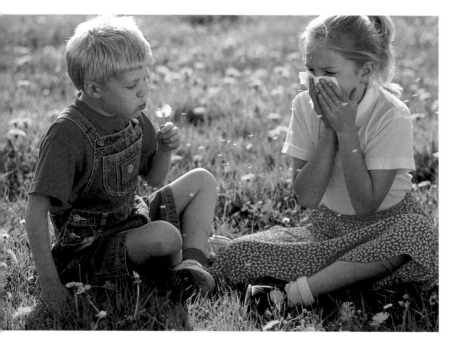

The pollen from certain types of grass or trees can cause an allergic skin reaction in some children, and often results in other symptoms, such as the sneezing and watery, itchy eyes of hay fever.

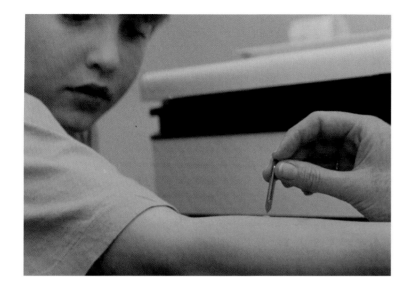

In a skin prick test, a drop of solution containing a potential allergen is placed on your child's skin. The skin is punctured with a needle, and if your child's system reacts to the allergen, a red, itchy wheal appears.

child may also have red, swollen and itchy eyes, or other symptoms such as headache, fatigue, joint pains, wheezing or fever. In severe cases, your child may experience breathing difficulties or a sudden drop in blood pressure. If your child has problems breathing or if he or she collapses, you should seek immediate medical help.

Allergy tests

The key to dealing with allergies is avoidance. But first you need to know what is causing your child's allergy. To help you identify or confirm the allergen, your doctor may arrange for your child to undergo some diagnostic tests. These include blood radioallergosorbent (RAST) testing — which involves taking a blood sample to measure the level of antibodies in your child's blood — and skin prick testing.

A number of other "allergy tests" are offered commercially, direct to the public. These include the antigen leukocyte cellular antibody test, hair analysis, autohomologous immune therapy, bioresonance diagnostics, electroacupuncture and vega testing. There is little scientific evidence that these tests are useful in diagnosing allergy. If in doubt, always take your child to see a doctor.

Contact dermatitis

This is the general term for a skin reaction resulting from direct contact between your child's skin and an external substance. Contact dermatitis can either be allergic or irritant, depending on whether the substance involved causes the type of allergic immune response described on p.22 or merely irritates your child's skin. Either type of contact dermatitis may result in your child's skin being inflamed, with red, blistering and itchy areas.

Common contact allergens include nickel (often found in jewelry), rubber (such as found in watch straps and elastic bands), many types of perfume and cosmetics, medications rubbed into the skin and some types of plants. Irritant contact dermatitis results from contact between your child's skin and irritating substances such as chemicals and detergents. The ammonia produced when urine reacts with the bacteria in feces is one very common irritant, often causing diaper rash in young children. See the potential irritants chart on pp.90–91 for further examples of substances that may be responsible.

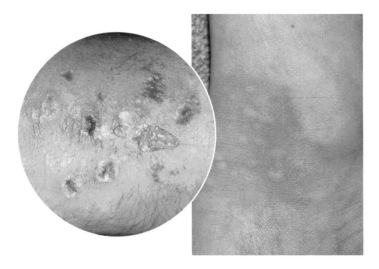

Itchy, raised welts (*left*), such as those caused by nettle rash, are a very common form of urticaria. More rarely, a severe urticaria rash (*far left*) may cause your child's skin to blister.

Treatment

In both forms of contact dermatitis, you should try to avoid contact between the offending substance and your child's skin, and care should be taken not to irritate your child's skin further — avoid using harsh soaps or detergents, or dressing your child in scratchy clothes. If you suspect a particular substance may be responsible, but you are not entirely sure, your doctor may wish to try a patch test on your child. This involves rubbing a suspect substance onto your child's skin, covering it, and inspecting it around 48 to 96 hours later.

Urticaria (hives, nettle rash)

This very common type of skin rash, with its distinctive red, itchy, raised wheals (hives), often results from some type of allergic reaction, although other, nonallergic reactions sometimes are responsible. It may be a form of contact dermatitis (see p.23), caused by direct skin contact with an irritant or allergen such as stinging nettles, but the rash also can be triggered by something your child has taken internally, such as a drug or food, or by some type of infection. In about half of cases the cause of the rash is never identified.

The onset of the rash is usually sudden, with widespread, bright-red skin, and often severe itching. Your child's skin also may blister. In some cases, other symptoms such as headache, fatigue, joint pains and fever may be present. In most cases the rash disappears within a few hours or days, but it may last longer: urticaria lasting less than six weeks is called acute, sudden or onset urticaria; if it lasts more than six weeks it is called chronic or recurrent urticaria.

Angioedema

Sometimes, urticaria may affect the deeper layers of your child's skin, causing more extensive swelling. This type of swelling is called angioedema and it can appear anywhere on your child's body. Most commonly it affects the mouth, tongue and eyelids. It may obstruct your child's breathing, in which case you should seek medical help immediately. Angioedema may be accompanied by a normal urticaria rash, or the two may occur separately.

Oral allergy syndrome

This is considered a form of contact urticaria that affects almost exclusively the mouth and throat. It is most commonly associated with eating fresh fruits and vegetables, and develops in some children with pollen allergies when the immune system fails to distinguish between pollen proteins and food proteins. It is nearly always preceded by hay fever. Symptoms include rapid onset of itching and swelling of the lips, tongue and throat. The symptoms generally resolve rapidly, but if your child's breathing is obstructed you should seek immediate medical help.

Causes of urticaria

Many different things can trigger your child's urticaria, and it is not always possible to identify a cause. Common stimuli include:

• **Foods**. Strawberries, seafood, fish, peanuts, milk, spices, tea, chocolate and eggs are all common troublemakers. These may be ingested, or the rash may result from direct skin contact, such as milk spilt on your child's skin.

• **Drugs**. Almost any drug can potentially cause your child to develop a rash. The most common cause of drug eruption is penicillin.

• **Infections**. Viral, fungal and even parasitic infections can all act as triggers.

• **Plants**. One of the most common culprits is the stinging nettle, although poison ivy can be very troublesome in some areas (see p.26).

THE **NATURAL** APPROACH

Broad-leafed dock plants, often found growing close to clumps of stinging nettles, have long been a popular remedy for nettle rash. To relieve the itching and burning caused by nettles, simply rub dock leaves over your child's skin at the site of the sting. Bear in mind that dock juice may irritate the skin if used too often.

• **Physical agents**. Exposure to sunlight, cold, heat or pressure all can cause a rash to develop.

See the potential irritants chart on pp. 90–91 for further information.

Treatment

Medical treatment is not usually necessary for mild or single occurrences. Antihistamines may help reduce your child's itching and any flushing by blocking the action of histamine, one of the chemicals that produces the allergic response (see p.22). You also can help relieve your child's itching by applying calamine lotion or a cold compress. If it is possible to identify the cause of the problem, encourage your child to avoid the offending substance in future.

For more serious or recurrent problems, it may be necessary to consult your doctor. To identify the cause of the urticaria, your doctor may want to consider the history of the rash, examine your child or carry out blood tests or allergy tests (see p.23). If no cause is found, he or she may suggest that you keep a food diary or put your child on an elimination diet (see p.85). A short course of prednisone (steroid) tablets may be given for severe episodes of urticaria that are unresponsive to antihistamines.

ALLERGIES

Poison oak, ivy and sumac

Found across many areas of the United States and southern Canada, these troublesome plants very commonly cause allergic contact dermatitis to unwary children. The plants contain a sap called urushiol, and if a child brushes against a damaged plant, he or she may experience a severe reaction starting with profound itching, and around 24 to 48 hours later (depending on sensitivity) an itchy, red, inflamed rash of small blisters. Not every child will come out in a rash on contact with the plants, but this is one rash where it is definitely better to be safe than sorry. The plants cause most problems during spring and summer.

Spotting the plants

Poison oak and poison ivy may appear either as shrubs or vines, and can be most easily recognized by their leaves, each of which contain three leaflets. The leaflets on poison ivy are pointed, generally oval-shaped, while those on poison oak are lobed. Poison oak also has hairy fruit, trunk and leaves. Poison sumac leaves have a row of 6 to 12 paired leaflets, with a further single leaflet at the end. All three plants have small, whitish berries in late summer or fall.

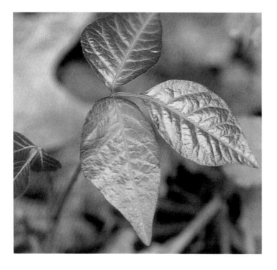

Treatment

Rinse your child's skin as soon as possible with plenty of cold running water. The sap may also be on your child's clothes, so these should also be washed. The rash will usually disappear within a week to 10 days, but may be extremely itchy while it lasts. Calamine lotion will help to soothe the itch. If your child has a severe rash, or rash with a fever, your doctor may prescribe a strong steroid cream.

Atopic eczema

This very common skin condition, sometimes called atopic dermatitis, affects around 1 in 10 children in North America, and usually develops in the first year of life (when it may also be called infantile eczema). Atopic eczema is a specific type of eczema, with strong hereditary tendencies and is possibly caused by some type of allergic reaction, which causes the skin to become more sensitive than usual to a variety of environmental factors. Most children have only mild irritation and will grow out of it, but if severe it can disrupt your child's quality of life.

Signs and symptoms

The skin of children affected by eczema is generally paler than that of others and tends to be very dry and sensitive. Eczema can appear anywhere, but usually begins with patches of dry, irritable, itchy skin on your child's face. It may then appear behind the ears and knees, and in the neck and elbow skin folds. Your child's skin may be red and inflamed with tiny pimples or blisters. The eczema may be moist and weeping, or your child's skin dry and thickened. The skin will be

To avoid a painful run-in with poison ivy (*left*), poison oak or poison sumac, it is worthwhile teaching your child the old adage, "leaves of three, let it be."

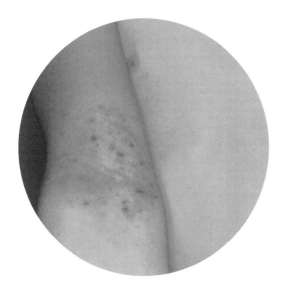

Atopic eczema often occurs in the skin folds, such as the elbow creases or behind the knees.

very itchy, and may scale or bleed. If your child's eczema is chronic — meaning it persists for a long time — scratching may eventually lead to thickening of your child's skin or lichenification. This is the body's internal defense mechanism to prevent further damage to the skin.

The extent of the rash varies from child to child. In severe cases, it may cover the whole body, and it may be more widespread at some times than others. A child with severe eczema is vulnerable to skin infections. Symptoms of an infection include a sudden worsening of the eczema, pus-filled spots, swollen glands and a raised temperature. Antibiotics may be needed. The herpes simplex (cold sore) virus can trigger a serious infection called eczema herpeticum, so it is important for anyone with a cold sore to avoid kissing a child with eczema.

Causes

The exact cause of atopic eczema is unknown, but it tends to run in families and is strongly associated with asthma and hay fever. Several factors may trigger the condition — these are known as precipitating factors — including the house dust mite, cat and dog hair, pollen, skin irritants such as wool and nylon material, detergents and soap and bubble baths.

Food allergy is commonly associated with eczema, but the part diet plays is complicated. Although research has found that many foods can trigger eczema, the most common being cow's milk, most children with atopic eczema do not react to foods. If your child has eczema, or it runs in the family, do not offer nuts, especially peanuts, until children are at least 3 years old, as these may trigger an allergic reaction.

Treatment of eczema

Always consult a doctor if you think that your child has eczema. Your doctor will be able to make a definite diagnosis and prescribe an appropriate treatment. The following treatments may help control or relieve the symptoms:

- **Emollients**. Eczema is a dry skin condition and the mainstay of treatment is to keep your child's skin soft and moist. Bathing alone can dry out the skin and ordinary soap should be used

HANDY **HINTS** ...

Parents often find the terms eczema and dermatitis confusing, and this is not surprising since the words are essentially synonymous. Dermatitis means an inflammation of the skin, and eczema — which comes from the Greek for "boiling out" — refers to the same thing. Both of the words are used to describe a range of conditions characterized by skin inflammation — contact dermatitis (see p.23) is a type of eczema, as is seborrheic dermatitis (see p.29).

ECZEMA AND DERMATITIS

sparingly or not at all. Instead, always use a suitable bath oil and apply emollients generously.

- **Steroid preparations**. If your child's skin becomes inflamed or infected, a steroid cream may be prescribed (see p.80). Steroids do not cure eczema, but they do accelerate the healing of badly damaged skin.
- **Antihistamines**. These may help to prevent itching and promote sleep, although some antihistamines cause daytime drowsiness.
- **Wet wraps**. Here, wet dressings are applied over the steroid cream and large amounts of emollients. The wraps cool your child's skin and can help break the scratch-itch cycle.

Other measures

Try to avoid exposing your child to irritants and allergens, particularly the house dust mite. Encase mattresses and pillows with nonallergenic bedding and wash bedclothes at 140°F (60°C) to kill the dust mite. Ban fluffy toys from the bedroom and if your child has a favorite toy, wash it once a week. Furnishings should be as simple as possible and dusting and vacuuming should be carried out frequently, preferably when your child is out of the room. Wooden or

THE **NATURAL** APPROACH

As with all treatments for eczema, complementary therapies will be effective for some children but not for others. It is important to use a properly qualified practitioner, and to inform your doctor of any treatment your child is having. Chinese herbal creams may be dangerous, as some have been found to contain excessive amounts of steroids (see p.84).

vinyl-covered floors are better than carpets. Do not let cats or dogs into your child's bedroom.

Whenever possible, dress your child in cotton clothing. Wool next to the skin can cause irritation and some man-made fibers prevent the skin breathing, and can make the eczema hot and itchy. Since hard water can make skin itchy, a water softener or water-softening agent may help. If your child is old enough, suggest he or she tries pinching itchy skin instead of scratching it.

Pityriasis alba

This is a common variant of atopic eczema, and appears as dry, scaly, white patches on a child's face. The patches often become more noticeable after exposure to sun, because the affected skin does not darken in the same way as the surrounding skin. Treatment is with emollients to keep the affected skin soft and moist.

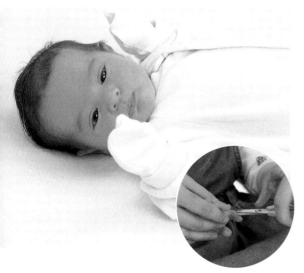

The itching caused by eczema can be intense, particularly at night. Keeping your child's nails trimmed short or covered with cotton mittens helps prevent further damage to sore skin.

rashes involving bacteria & fungi

Seborrheic dermatitis

This common, but noninfectious, rash — sometimes called seborrheic eczema — usually affects children at around 2 months of age. The exact cause is unclear. Seborrhea means an excessive oiliness of the skin, and in some types of seborrheic dermatitis, such as cradle cap (see p.17), this may be enough to cause inflammation. However, it is thought that this excess sebum can sometimes cause an overgrowth of yeastlike fungi, called pityrosporum, that also contribute to the irritation of your child's skin.

What to look for

There may be thick, crusted scales on your baby's scalp, similar to cradle cap, with redness or inflammation. A red, scaly rash may spread to your child's face and body — especially the forehead, eyebrows and behind the ears. The dermatitis may also occur in the diaper area, causing an inflamed and flaky skin rash with small, white skin scales, which may spread up your baby's abdomen. Parents may sometimes confuse the rash with atopic eczema (see p.26) — see a doctor if you are unsure of the diagnosis.

Treatment

In mild cases, treat your child's scalp as for cradle cap (see p.17). In addition, you should bathe your child daily, using a nonsoap product such as emulsifying cream. This will loosen the scales and moisturize your child's skin. Pat the skin dry after bathing, and reapply an oil-free moisturizing cream several times a day. If the rash is severe or infected, you should see a doctor. A mild hydrocortisone cream, or a combination cream with hydrocortisone and an antifungal agent, may be needed.

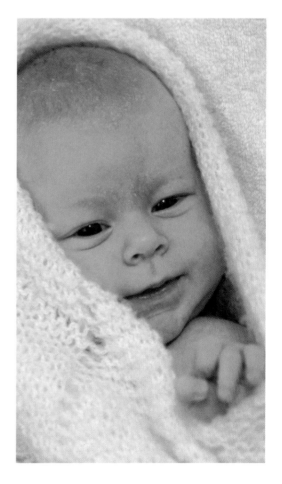

The rash caused by seborrheic dermatitis may look sore, but it does not harm your baby, and probably will bother you more than your child.

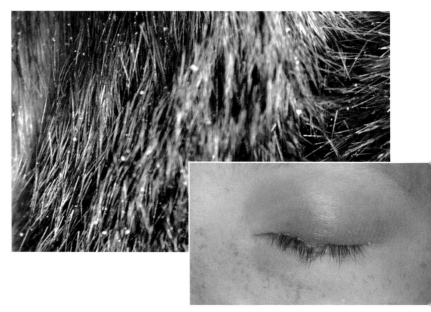

Microorganisms play a role in both dandruff (*top right*) and cellulitis. But while the yeastlike organisms that cause dandruff are largely harmless, facial cellulitis (*bottom right*) is a potentially serious bacterial infection.

Dandruff

Mild scaling and shedding of skin cells on the scalp, without any redness, is usually classified as dandruff, while more severe scaling is referred to as seborrheic dermatitis (see p.29). Dandruff is caused primarily by the same excess sebum and yeastlike organisms that are responsible for seborrheic dermatitis, although other factors — such as hair products or sun exposure — can sometimes play a part.

If your child has dandruff, you will be able to see white flakes in his or her hair, as well as on the collar or shoulders of clothes. This common condition tends to start in adolescence and is not the same as cradle cap (see p.17), a similar flaking of the scalp in young babies.

Treatment

To treat your child's dandruff, shampoo his or her hair using a gentle shampoo, three to four times a week for three to four weeks. Rinse well after shampooing. If your child's dandruff does not clear, try a mild, medicated shampoo suitable for children. Antidandruff shampoos may be harsh on your child's hair, so don't forget to apply conditioner after shampooing. If the

medicated shampoo is not effective after three to four weeks, if your child's dandruff is severe or if there is any redness or irritation, you should take your child to see a doctor.

Cellulitis

Many different types of bacteria inhabit your child's skin, but because the skin provides such an effective barrier, these microorganisms are usually harmless. Occasionally, however, an injury — such as a cut, wound or burn — allows these bacteria to enter your child's skin. This may result in cellulitis — an acute (sudden) infection of the soft tissues underneath the skin. The affected area will be red, hot, swollen and tender to the touch. Your child will also feel unwell and have fever and chills.

Cellulitis may affect your child's face, eyes, scalp, neck, legs or anus. Specific symptoms of facial cellulitis may include a respiratory tract infection, vomiting and loss of appetite. The swelling may advance to the front of the neck causing swallowing difficulties. Cellulitis occurring around the eye (orbital cellulitis) may

CELLULITIS

cause swelling of your child's eyelid and pain or tenderness in his or her eye, headache, sickness and a watery discharge from your child's nose. Symptoms of perianal cellulitis include redness around the anal region, pain when passing stools, blood-stained stools and itching.

Treatment

Take your child to see a doctor. The usual treatment for cellulitis is intensive antibiotic treatment, usually with penicillin, so make sure your doctor knows if your child is allergic to this. To lessen your child's pain and discomfort, you may wish to give him or her a nonaspirin analgesic such as acetaminophen or ibuprofen, or apply a cool compress. In severe cases, your child may need hospitalization.

Erysipelas

This is a severe form of cellulitis caused by streptococci bacteria, and most commonly affects the face or lower leg. Erysipelas often occurs when your child is already suffering from a streptococcal sore throat, since the presence of the bacteria make it more likely that your child will also pick up the skin infection. It starts suddenly, with high fever, headache, a chill and

vomiting. An itchy, inflamed and painful, bright-red patch appears on your child's skin. Vesicles or blisters appear on the skin surface, burst and then crust over. You may also be able to feel enlarged, tender lymph nodes under your child's skin as his or her body attempts to fight the infection. Treatment is the same as for other forms of cellulitis (see p.30).

Erythema multiforme

It is not always quite clear what causes this skin rash, although it is usually triggered by a viral or bacterial infection, especially by the herpes simplex (cold sore) virus. In other cases there may be no obvious cause, although it is possible that the rash may occur as a reaction to certain medications. The rash is characterized by round, raised skin lesions, which often have a central blister, lending them a bull's-eye appearance. There may be a variety of lesions, including macules (discolorations level with the skin surface), papules (small solid lumps) or bullae (large, raised, fluid-filled blisters). The rash may occur at any age and is more common in boys than in girls. It will usually clear on its own, but you should contact a doctor if your child becomes feverish or unwell.

Raised lesions with a characteristic targetlike shape are the most distinctive feature of erythema multiforme.

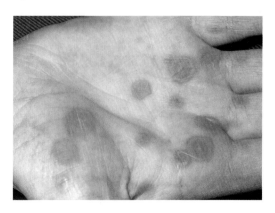

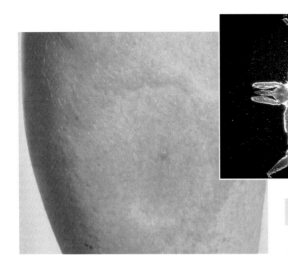

In most cases, the first sign of Lyme disease is a large, red, spreading rash (*far left*), forming around the site of a bite from an infected deer tick (*left*).

HEALTH **ALERT** ...

Early diagnosis of Lyme disease is very important, as the fever, muscle aches and fatigue of Lyme disease can easily be mistaken for viral infections such as influenza, while joint pain can be mistaken for other types of arthritis, such as rheumatoid arthritis. If your child experiences any of the symptoms in the month or so following a tick bite, you should always remember to inform your doctor of the bite.

LYME DISEASE

Lyme disease

This is an infection caused by the bite of a deer tick infected with the *Borrelia burgdorferi* bacterium. The condition was first named in 1975, after an outbreak of arthritis associated with tick bites near Lyme, Connecticut. Since then, reports have increased dramatically, and it has become an important public health problem in some areas of the United States. Lyme disease is most prevalent in children under 15 years old and adults older than 29.

If diagnosed early enough, Lyme disease is easily treatable with antibiotics, but it is often difficult to diagnose because its symptoms and signs mimic those of many other diseases. If left untreated, the disease may develop over months or years, causing nervous system abnormalities including numbness, pain and Bell's palsy (paralysis of the facial muscles). Meningitis and arthritis symptoms may also occur.

Signs and symptoms

The disease may first show itself as a red, circular rash (erythema migrans) in the area of the tick bite, usually developing between 3 to 30 days after the bite. The patch then expands, often to a large size. Sometimes many patches appear, varying in shape. Common sites are the thigh, groin, trunk and armpits. The center of the rash may clear as it enlarges, resulting in a bull's-eye appearance. The rash may be warm, but it usually is not painful. Early symptoms may resemble influenza, with swollen glands near the site of the tick bite, headaches, muscle and joint pain, chills and fever, and tiredness.

Prevention

If you know that your child will be walking through tick-infested areas, you should perform daily tick checks. Try to remove an attached tick within 72 hours. Using tweezers, grasp the tick as close to the skin surface as possible and pull straight back with a slow, steady force. Avoid crushing the tick's body.

other noncontagious rashes

Psoriasis

Children with this condition suffer from an excessive production of new skin cells — about 10 times faster than normal — while the speed at which the old cells are shed remains normal. As a result, the new skin cells accumulate, and produce inflamed, thick, red or pink-colored patches. Psoriasis is not infectious and does not usually itch, but it can cause your child physical discomfort and embarrassment.

The underlying cause of psoriasis is unknown. It tends to run in families and is less common in black children, so it is likely that sufferers have some type of genetic predisposition. It can be triggered by external factors such as infection (particularly a throat infection), trauma, stress or medications. The peak age of onset in children is 10 years and it rarely occurs before the age of 2. Occasionally, children with psoriasis develop chronic arthritis.

Recognizing common types

There are several different types of psoriasis. The most likely type in children is guttate psoriasis, with numerous, small, scaly, light-pink to red patches resembling drops of water. An attack usually resolves over three to four months. Some children may develop the chronic plaque variety. This manifests as raised pink or red patches with sharply defined edges, covered in silvery scales. The patches range in size from tiny "plaques" to far more extensive areas.

Treatment

Although it cannot be completely cured, there are various treatments available to help keep your child's psoriasis under control, including:
- **Emollients**. These help to descale your child's skin and prevent drying and cracking.
- **Coal tar products**. The anti-inflammatory and antiscaling properties of coal tar may offer

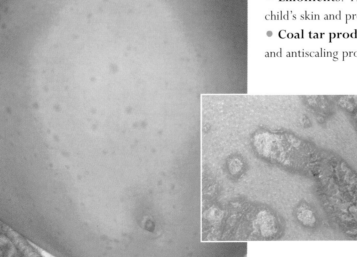

Chronic plaque psoriasis (*left*) may affect any part of your child's body, but is most common on the elbows, knees and scalp. Guttate psoriasis (*far left*) is more usually found across your child's trunk and upper limbs.

your child relief, although it can be smelly or messy. Coal tar may be used with other ingredients such as coconut oil or salicylic acid.

- **Sunlight or ultraviolet lamp**. UV light may help relieve your child's psoriasis, although sunburn will make the rash worse.
- **Topical steroids**. These can be useful in reducing inflamed or sore psoriasis, but extensive use can have side effects (see p.80).
- **Salicylic acid**. This helps to reduce scaling and is usually used in conjunction with other preparations, such as dithranol.
- **Dithranol**. This well-established treatment works by slowing down skin-cell division. It can cause burning and irritation, or stain the skin.
- **Vitamin D derivatives**. Medications such as calcipotriol or tacalcitol are very effective treatments for psoriasis, but can cause burning and irritation. These medications can interfere with your child's uptake of calcium.

Pityriasis rosea

This common condition usually affects young adults or adolescents, but sometimes also younger children, and begins with a pink, scaly, oval "herald patch." Initially it may appear to be a fungal infection, such as ringworm (see p.39). Occasionally, the patch does not appear at all. A secondary eruption appears 2 to 21 days after the appearance of the herald patch. Multiple small, flat, round or oval-shaped, pink or salmon-colored spots appear on the child's trunk and spread along his or her thighs and arms. Spots on the trunk have been described as resembling a Christmas-tree pattern. More rarely, spots appear on the hands, face and feet. The lesions themselves do not usually produce discomfort, although many children complain of itching. Some children also suffer from a mild fever, fatigue, headache or pain in the joints. Oral lesions can also occur.

The exact cause of the rash is still unknown: it is thought to result from a viral infection, but this has not been proven. The rash is self-limiting and generally clears in six to eight weeks, although it can last for as long as five months.

Treatment

If you suspect your child has pityriasis rosea, treatment is not normally required — the rash is self-limiting and is not usually irritating. If it is itchy, your child may benefit from emollients, mild topical corticosteroid creams or other medications to control the itching. Ultraviolet light (UVB) phototherapy may also help decrease the severity of the disease.

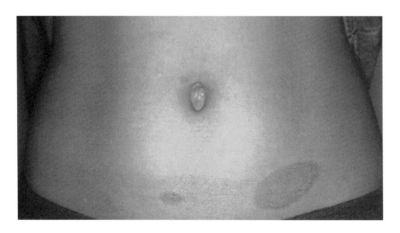

A distinctive oval-shaped patch, typically located on your child's trunk, usually "heralds" the arrival of pityriasis rosea.

Acne

Almost all children suffer the embarrassment of acne at some point in their lives, with problems usually starting at, or just after puberty. It may occasionally start as early as 8 years of age, and sometimes can affect infants (see p.17). Acne occurs when the sebaceous (oil-producing) glands, which normally keep your child's hair and skin lubricated, produce too much oily sebum. This increased production can cause a blockage of the hair follicles, causing bacteria and dead skin cells to build up, and resulting in acne spots. Acne most commonly occurs after puberty because it is around then that rising levels of hormones, called androgens, stimulate your child's sebaceous glands. Acne tends to run in families, and there is no evidence that eating fatty foods, or too much candy or chocolate can cause acne. Neither is it caused by poor hygiene.

Symptoms

The face is most commonly affected, but acne can also occur on the neck, back and chest. The number and type of lesions can vary enormously, depending on the type and severity of your child's acne. Lesions may be inflamed or noninflamed.

● **Noninflamed acne** consists of blackheads and whiteheads. Blackheads (open comedones) contain a tiny plug of sebum and a collection of skin pigment melanin — the "black" of the blackhead is melanin, not dirt. Whiteheads (closed comedones) are similar, but skin-colored.

● **Inflamed lesions,** which contain pus, include red spots (papules), yellow spots (pustules), large, deep spots (nodules) and cysts (swellings filled with fluid). In severe acne, the deep-seated spots may damage the underlying skin tissue as they heal, and cause scarring. Scars may appear as small, depressed pits; sharp, steep-sided depressions known as ice-pick scars; or raised keloid scars (see p.68).

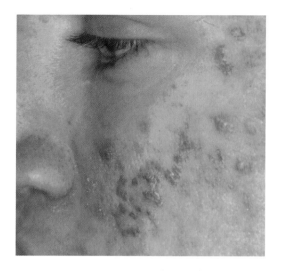

Severe acne can sometimes cause scarring, especially if your child picks at or squeezes the spots, so try to persuade your child to resist the temptation.

Treatment

Make sure your child washes his or her face twice a day with a mild soap. Exposure to sunlight, without getting sunburnt, may help. Mild acne can be treated by over-the-counter preparations, but a doctor should be consulted in moderate or severe cases. There are two basic forms of treatment for acne: topical treatments (applied directly to the skin) and oral treatments, which can be prescribed only by a doctor. In some cases, both topical and oral medications will be used. To keep acne from spreading, apply topical medications about half an inch around the

THE **NATURAL** APPROACH

The powerful antiseptic properties of tea tree oil make it an effective alternative to other topical treatments. Dab the oil on spots and comedones, or use the oil in a tea tree face wash.

affected area. You will need to be persistent — it may be several months before your child's skin shows any signs of improvement.

- **Mild acne**. If your child has only a few comedones and spots, and little inflammation, it may be sufficient to use a topical preparation at the site of the acne. Anti-inflammatory and antibacterial washes or gels, such as those containing benzoyl peroxide, iodine or vitamin A derivatives called retinoids, can be used directly on the problem areas.
- **Moderate acne**. For more inflamed papules and pustules, and if topical antibiotics fail to have an effect, your child may be prescribed oral antibiotics such as tetracycline.
- **Severe acne**. If there are numerous, inflamed pustules, nodules and cysts, which risk causing scarring, your child should see a dermatologist (skin specialist). Girls may be prescribed an antiandrogen and contraceptive preparation. Oral isotretinoin, a powerful antiacne drug that is sometimes prescribed in severe cases, is very effective but may cause serious side effects.

Benzoyl peroxide

Both comedones and inflamed lesions respond well to benzoyl peroxide, which has keratolytic (encouraging the removal of dead skin cells) and antibacterial properties. It is available in a range of creams, lotions and gels, both by prescription and over the counter, and is safe for both adults and children to use. Its disadvantage is that it may bleach clothes, irritate your child's skin or cause excessive dryness. It may take two to three weeks before you begin to see signs of improvement. Benzoyl peroxide can also be combined with topical antibiotics (see box, above). Products containing benzoyl peroxide include Benzac, Brevoxyl, PanOxyl and Triaz.

COMMON **MEDICATIONS** ...

FOR ACNE

Retinoids and topical antibiotics are suitable treatments for mild to moderate acne. The medications given here are available by prescription only, although some topical antibiotics are available to buy over the counter.

Retinoids
Retin-A (active ingredient, tretinoin)
Isotrex (active ingredient, isotretinoin)
Differin (active ingredient, adapalene)

Topical antibiotics
Benzamycin (active ingredients, benzoyl peroxide and erythromycin)
Cleocin T/Dalacin T (active ingredient, clindamycin)

Retinoids

Chemical derivatives of vitamin A, called retinoids, are particularly effective in treating noninflamed comedonal acne. The disadvantage of retinoids such as tretinoin and isotretinoin is that there may be some scaling, irritation and redness. They may also make your child's skin vulnerable to irritation from sunlight. New products containing adapalene, which causes fewer side effects, have recently become available. Retinoids are available only by prescription (see box, above) and they are not suitable for children under the age of 12.

3 Contagious rashes

Infectious diseases are a common feature of childhood, and many of these infections result in some type of skin rash. Because contagious rashes are usually spread from child to child, through contact with someone who has the infection, schools and child-care centers are the ideal places for them to spread.

The majority of contagious rashes are caused by viruses, although fungal infections such as athlete's foot are also very common, and bacterial infections produce some serious childhood diseases, including impetigo, scarlet fever and bacterial meningitis.

Thanks to immunization, some serious infectious diseases, including measles, mumps and rubella, are now uncommon in developed countries. They are not eliminated, however, and a reduction in the number of children being immunized could see epidemics reemerge. And for many other infectious rashes, vaccines are not yet available to protect your child.

FUNGAL INFECTIONS athlete's foot

CONTAGIOUS UNTIL SYMPTOMS DISAPPEAR

COMMON

unknown
INCUBATION PERIOD

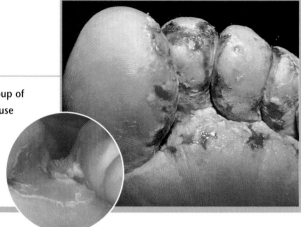

➡ This common infection is caused by a group of fungi called the dermatophytes, which also cause ringworm (see p.39). Known medically as tinea pedis, it occurs mostly in adolescents and adults, but can be picked up by younger children.

What to look for ...

1 Itching and burning of the skin between the toes, especially the fourth and fifth toes.
2 Peeling or scaling of the skin, which may turn "soggy" and white.
3 A scaly, red rash, which may also spread to the soles of the feet. If untreated, the skin may crack or bleed.
★ Pus-filled sores or ulcers sometimes result from an accompanying bacterial infection.

What to do ...

1 Wash your child's feet once or twice daily and dry thoroughly, especially between the toes, and remove dead skin or tissue with a tissue or paper towel.
2 After washing, apply an antifungal cream, spray or powder. Symptoms may take two to three weeks to disappear. Treatment should be continued for at least one week after the symptoms have disappeared.
3 Socks should be changed daily. If possible, use those made from natural fibers and let your child wear open-toed shoes or sandals. Sneakers or shoes made from synthetic

materials that don't allow the feet to breathe should not be worn for prolonged periods.
4 See your doctor if the infection persists or there is a discharge.
★ Current evidence suggests 1 percent terbinafine cream is one of the most effective topical treatments (see p.78). If a topical treatment fails or the infection is widespread, oral antifungal medication may be prescribed.

Take note ...

✎ The infection thrives in warm, moist conditions. To prevent infection, encourage your child to wear flip-flops in communal changing places such as swimming pools.
✎ Don't let your child share towels, or wear socks or shoes belonging to others.

THE **NATURAL** APPROACH

Natural remedies for treating athlete's foot include garlic juice — a powerful antifungal agent — and tea tree oil.

ringworm

   variable

CONTAGIOUS FOR AS LONG AS LESIONS PERSIST UNCOMMON CALL YOUR DOCTOR INCUBATION PERIOD

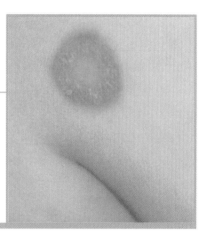

 This infection has nothing to do with worms: like athlete's foot, it is caused by a group of fungi called the dermatophytes, and is known as ringworm because the infections tend to form wormlike round patches with smooth centers. Ringworm may occur on the scalp (tinea capitis), body (tinea corporis) or, more rarely, the nails (tinea unguium).

What to look for ...

scalp ringworm

1 A round, scaly, itchy bald patch, with stumps of broken hairs of variable length, on the scalp. Breakage of hairs at their roots causes the appearance referred to as black-dot tinea capitis.

2 A raised, inflamed boggy mass, called a kerion, which may develop from the patch.

body ringworm

Ringlike patches with a red, itchy, scaly edge, which may sometimes have vesicles. The most common site is the trunk. As the ringworm spreads, the center of the patch often clears to leave normal skin.

nail ringworm

Discolored, thick and brittle nails.

What to do ...

1 CALL YOUR DOCTOR, who may examine scalp ringworm under ultraviolet light (Wood's light) filtered through a special glass, to determine the type of fungus causing the infection. Some types will glow green under the light.

★ Your doctor will also take samples of skin scrapings, plucked hairs or nail clippings and send these to the laboratory to identify the type of fungus before starting treatment.

★ Your doctor may prescribe an oral antifungal medication (griseofulvin) for scalp and body ringworm, to be used for at least six weeks. A topical antifungal cream may also be given for body ringworm. For nail ringworm, griseofulvin should be taken for at least six months.

2 Give your child his or her own hairbrush, comb and towel.

Take note ...

✎ Ringworm may be caught from another person, from animals or from the soil.

✎ Scalp ringworm occurs mainly in children. It spreads easily from person to person and during epidemics may affect 10 percent to 20 percent of susceptible children. It is rare after the age of puberty.

BACTERIAL INFECTIONS impetigo

HIGHLY CONTAGIOUS

FAIRLY COMMON

CALL YOUR DOCTOR

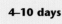

4–10 days

INCUBATION PERIOD

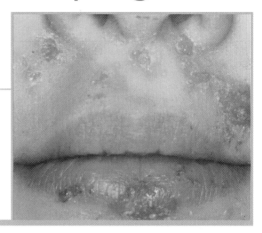

This highly infectious skin disease may be caused by either the bacteria *Staphylococcus aureus* or *Streptococcus*, or a mixture of both. Impetigo spreads rapidly by direct contact or through sharing infected towels and washcloths.

What to look for ...

1 Tender red spots. The most common site is on the face, particularly around the mouth and nose, but other areas such as the chest and hands can be infected.
2 Blisters, which develop from the spots and then burst, exuding a yellow, sticky liquid.
3 Golden-colored crusts, over a red, weeping area, forming when the lesions dry.

What to do ...

1 CALL YOUR DOCTOR. Impetigo must be treated quickly as it is infectious and spreads rapidly. In mild cases, your doctor will prescribe a topical antibiotic cream (fusidic acid or mupirocin). Before applying the cream, your doctor may recommend soaking the crust in a saline (salt) solution or antiseptic. In severe cases, an oral or injectible antibiotic may be prescribed.
2 Wash loose crusts gently two to three times a day with soap and water and pat dry with a paper towel. Give your child a separate washcloth and towel, and boil or machine wash at a high temperature after use.
3 Encourage your child not to scratch or pick at the blisters.
4 Keep your child away from school until the lesions are healed.

Take note ...

✎ Impetigo most commonly affects children under the age of 10, and is the most common bacterial skin infection in children.
✎ It can occur in both healthy skin or as a secondary infection in skin that is damaged, for example, by eczema, scabies or by a cut.
✎ In newborns and young infants, impetigo may cause large blisters (bullae) on the buttocks, trunk and face.
✎ Unless hygiene measures are taken, impetigo can spread rapidly through a family or a school.
✎ In a few children, staphylococci bacteria can cause a life-threatening toxic reaction where the epidermis layer of the skin peels off in sheets (staphylococcal scalded skin syndrome). If you think your child is suffering from this reaction, you should call a doctor immediately.

scarlet fever

  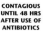

2–7 days

CONTAGIOUS
UNTIL 48 HRS
AFTER USE OF
ANTIBIOTICS

FAIRLY
COMMON

CALL YOUR
DOCTOR

INCUBATION PERIOD

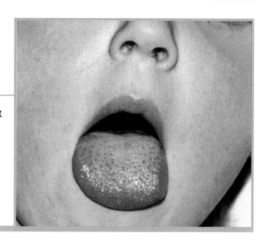

➡ Caused by Group A streptococci bacteria, this throat infection produces a toxin that causes a rash in sensitive persons. It is spread by inhalation of infected droplets coughed or sneezed into the air. Previously a dangerous disease, since the advent of antibiotics, scarlet fever is both less common and less severe.

What to look for ...

1 Sore throat or tonsillitis, headache and a high fever. The tonsils and back of the throat may be covered with a white coating, or be red and swollen and contain pus.

2 A white coating on the tongue, with red spots protruding ("the white strawberry tongue"). Four or five days later, the coating peels off, leaving a bright-red appearance ("the red strawberry tongue").

3 A rash, which starts as tiny, dark red bumps the size of pinheads. It usually develops on the neck and face. The face and forehead become red but the area around the mouth remains pale. The rash then travels to the rest of the body. When pressed, the rash usually blanches (turns white).

4 Peeling skin, especially on the hands and feet, which may occur as the rash fades.

What to do ...

1 CALL YOUR DOCTOR, who may take a swab from your child's throat in order to culture the bacteria in the laboratory and confirm that it is a streptococcal infection before giving antibiotics.

2 Let your child rest, give him or her plenty of fluids and a nonaspirin medication such as acetaminophen or ibuprofen for the sore throat and to reduce the fever.

3 If eating is painful, give your child soft foods such as ice cream or yogurt, or liquids such as nutritious soups or milkshakes.

Take note ...

✎ Antibiotics will help to prevent any risk of rare complications from streptococci such as rheumatic disease or kidney inflammation.

✎ Streptococci bacteria may also cause impetigo (see p.40).

✎ Children may be the carriers of streptococci bacteria without having any obvious symptoms.

Kawasaki disease

POSSIBLY CONTAGIOUS (CAUSE UNKNOWN)

RARE

CALL YOUR DOCTOR

unknown

INCUBATION PERIOD

➜ Kawasaki disease is an illness that can affect the blood vessels of the heart and result in complications such as heart attacks, heart failure and coronary artery thrombosis. The exact cause is still unknown, although it is believed to be caused by an infectious agent, such as bacteria.

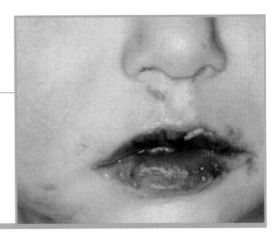

What to look for ...

1 A high fever, above 102°F (39°C), lasting five days or more without clear explanation, and at least four of the following:

2 Conjunctivitis (an eye infection causing red eyes).

3 A red rash, generally occuring in the groin or trunk area.

4 Red, dry, cracked lips, which may also be accompanied by a strawberry-colored tongue or a red, infected throat and mouth.

5 Changes to the hands and feet, such as redness or swelling of the fingers or toes. Peeling skin on the hands, feet or groin may appear 14 to 21 days into the illness.

6 Swelling of the glands in the neck.

What to do ...

CALL YOUR DOCTOR. An early diagnosis is important to help prevent the risk of fatal heart complications. There is no laboratory test for Kawasaki disease, but if the signs suggest the disease is the cause of your child's illness, the doctor will want to admit him or her to the hospital immediately.

★ Treatment will include a high dose of immunoglobulin, given to your child intravenously (through a vein) to lower the risk of coronary complications. A high dose of aspirin will also be given to reduce the risk of complications such as thrombosis.

Take note ...

✎ Treatment usually results in rapid improvement. Very rarely, if the disease causes serious heart problems, it may be necessary for children to undergo surgery. Complications such as arthritis, meningitis or diarrhea may also occur.

✎ There is a 1 percent to 2 percent chance of recurrence, which may occur years later.

✎ Kawasaki disease was first reported in Japanese children in 1967 and there appears to be a higher incidence in Asian and Afro-Caribbean children. However, the disease is found worldwide.

✎ Kawasaki disease mainly affects children under the age of 5, with the peak incidence at the end of the first year of life, and is more common in boys than girls.

meningitis & septicemia

2–10 days

CONTAGIOUS
UNTIL BACTERIA
DISAPPEAR FROM
BODY

UNCOMMON

CALL YOUR
DOCTOR

INCUBATION PERIOD

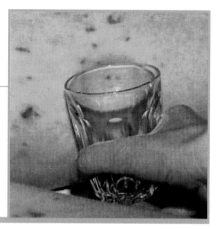

 Meningitis is a dangerous inflammation of the meninges (the fine membranes lining the brain and spinal cord) caused by a viral or bacterial infection. Meningococcal, one of the most common types of bacterial meningitis, often develops together with septicemia (blood poisoning). This can also develop on its own, and in either case may be life-threatening.

What to look for ...

Signs, which may not all be present and may appear in any order, include:

meningitis

1 A high temperature, vomiting, headache or stiff neck. Your baby or child may be drowsy or confused and dislike bright lights.
2 In babies, a fever, a high-pitched, shrill or moaning cry, a bulging fontanelle (soft spot on the head), a staring expression, an arching of the back or a floppy body.
3 A rash, which may start as a cluster of tiny blood spots that look like pinpricks, and develops into large purple marks. The rash does not blanch (turn white) under pressure.

septicemia

1 A more extensive rash, which does not blanch under pressure. This may appear anywhere on the body, and starts as pin-prick red spots, which quickly develop into large purple marks, like fresh bruises.
2 Vomiting, fever with cold hands and feet, fast breathing or joint, muscle or abdominal pain. The child may become unconscious.
★ In septicemia without meningitis, stiff neck, headache and dislike of bright lights may be absent, but the rash may be extensive.
★ Under fives and teens are particularly vulnerable to meningitis and septicemia.
★ A rash is not present in all cases of meningitis and septicemia. If present, the disease is in an advanced stage.

What to do ...

1 Try the "tumbler test." If your child has pinprick red spots or large purple marks, press a glass tumbler against them to see if they fade or turn white under pressure.
2 MENINGITIS AND SEPTICEMIA ARE MEDICAL EMERGENCIES. If you suspect your child has meningitis or septicemia, or if the rash does not fade or turn white under pressure, CONTACT YOUR DOCTOR URGENTLY or take your child to the nearest emergency department.
★ The doctor may give your child an injection of benzylpenicillin to halt the disease, and admit him or her to hospital.

VIRAL INFECTIONS measles

7–12 days

HIGHLY
CONTAGIOUS
UNTIL FOUR DAYS
AFTER RASH
APPEARS

UNCOMMON

CALL YOUR
DOCTOR

INCUBATION PERIOD

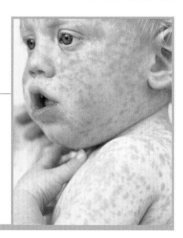

➡ This dangerous, highly infectious disease, sometimes called rubeola, is caused by the rubeola virus. Spread by droplet infection, measles was very common until the 1960s when a vaccine was first developed. The MMR immunization program means that it is more rare today, but outbreaks still occur in areas where immunization levels drop. Babies in the first 6 to 8 months of life usually have a natural immunity from their mothers.

What to look for ...

1 Severe coldlike symptoms. Your child may feel miserable and unwell.

2 A rash of brownish pink spots, which appears three to four days later, starting behind the ears. The rash spreads down over the face, neck, trunk and limbs over three days. It fades in the same order as it appears. The spots may merge to form blotches.

3 Small white spots (Koplik's spots), similar to grains of salt, which may be seen inside the mouth one to two days before the rash.

★ Some children also experience swollen lymph glands or sensitivity to light.

What to do ...

1 CALL YOUR DOCTOR. Although measles is a viral infection, the doctor may prescribe antibiotics for any secondary bacterial infection or complications.

2 Keep your child cool and well rested, and give him or her plenty of clear fluids.

3 Give your child a nonaspirin, fever-reducing medicine such as acetaminophen or ibuprofen, to bring the temperature down.

Take note ...

✎ Complications occur in about 1 in 15 children. These may include otitis media (middle ear infection), pneumonia, bronchitis and convulsions. Encephalitis, a potentially life-threatening inflammation of the brain cells, occurs in around 1 in 5,000 cases. Children with a chronic illness or those with Down's syndrome are at particular risk from complications.

✎ All children are offered protection against measles as part of the measles, mumps and rubella (MMR) immunization program, usually at 12 to 15 months with a second dose between 3 and 5 years of age as part of the preschool booster program.

THE **NATURAL** APPROACH

Add a few drops of camomile or lavender oil to the bath water to soothe your child, and help him or her to sleep (see p.86).

rubella

    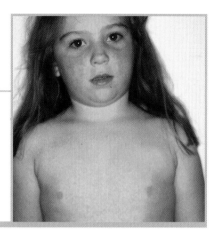

CONTAGIOUS UNTIL ONE WEEK AFTER RASH APPEARS	UNCOMMON	CALL YOUR DOCTOR	**14–21 days** INCUBATION PERIOD	DANGEROUS TO FETUS

➡ Commonly called German measles, this is normally a mild, infectious disease, caused by the rubella virus. It is most common in children aged between 4 and 9 who have not been immunized against rubella. If rubella occurs in a woman during the first 16 weeks of pregnancy, it may affect her unborn child.

What to look for …

1 A mild fever, lasting for one or two days, and swollen glands behind the ears.

2 A rash of tiny, pink, slightly raised spots which begins behind the ears, or on the face. This rash then spreads downward over the rest of the body.

★ Other symptoms may include swollen glands in other parts of the body, conjunctivitis, sore throat, headache and, occasionally, pain and swelling in the joints.

What to do …

1 Keep infected children away from pregnant women.

2 To reduce any fever or discomfort, give your child a nonaspirin medication such as acetaminophen or ibuprofen.

3 CALL YOUR DOCTOR if your child develops a high temperature, a severe headache, is drowsy or otherwise appears ill, or if you are in early pregnancy and have not already had a blood test to check that you have immunity.

Take note …

✎ THE RUBELLA VIRUS CAN AFFECT A DEVELOPING FETUS. Rubella infection in a mother in the first 16 weeks of pregnancy can cause congenital rubella syndrome with serious malformations, or even death to her fetus. After 16 weeks' gestation, fetal damage is rare. Before a first pregnancy, a woman of child-bearing age should have a blood test to confirm she is immune to rubella. This test measures the amount of rubella antibodies present in the blood.

✎ To prevent rubella, all children are offered immunization as part of the measles, mumps and rubella (MMR) immunization program, usually at 12 to 15 months with a second dose between 3 and 5 years as part of the preschool booster program.

fifth disease

  2–4 weeks

CONTAGIOUS
UNTIL RASH
APPEARS

FAIRLY
COMMON

INCUBATION PERIOD

DANGEROUS
TO FETUS

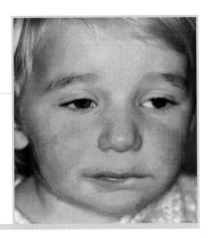

➡ Also called slapped cheek syndrome, since it is characterized by bright-red, slaplike patches on the cheeks, or erythema infectiosum, this is caused by the parvovirus B19. The virus is spread from person to person from fluids in the mouth and throat, especially when someone who has the virus coughs or sneezes. It is most common in children between 5 and 10, but it can occur in adults.

What to look for ...

1 Mild fever and coldlike symptoms (sore throat, slight fever, headache, pink eyes, fatigue, itching and nasal discharge).

2 Bright-red, warm, raised patches like slap marks, which appear on both cheeks around a week later.

3 A lacy, pink, slightly raised rash that spreads to the arms, trunk, thighs and buttocks, and which may come and go for up to three weeks.

★ Rarely, an older child may have joint pains.

What to do ...

1 Keep your child cool and well hydrated.

2 If your child is suffering from headache, pain or discomfort, give him or her a nonaspirin medication such as acetaminophen or ibuprofen.

★ No other treatment is usually necessary. The rash causes no discomfort and should eventually disappear.

★ Your child is not infectious once the rash appears, so there is no need to keep him or her away from others.

Take note ...

✎ Fifth disease is most common in children between 5 and 10, but can occur in adults.

✎ The rash may appear briefly if your child becomes heated or chilled, or spends time in the sun.

✎ PARVOVIRUS B19 CAN AFFECT A DEVELOPING FETUS. Most pregnant women will be immune, but if you, or anyone else who is pregnant, has been in contact with the virus or develops a rash, contact your doctor immediately.

✎ Parvovirus B19 temporarily suppresses the production of red blood cells, so children with chronic hemolytic anemia such as sickle cell anemia or thalassemia may suffer an aplastic crisis (become severely anemic). Children who have an immune deficiency disease may become seriously ill. CALL YOUR DOCTOR if you think your child may be at risk.

✎ Fifth disease is easily confused with other viral rashes or a medication-related rash. If in doubt, contact your doctor or pharmacist.

chickenpox

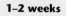

CONTAGIOUS UNTIL LAST BLISTER CRUSTS OVER	**VERY COMMON**	**CALL YOUR DOCTOR**	**1–2 weeks** INCUBATION PERIOD	**DANGEROUS TO FETUS**

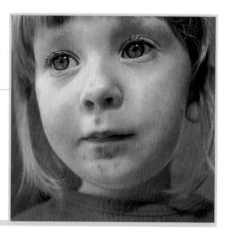

➲ Caused by the varicella-zoster virus and known medically as varicella, chickenpox is highly contagious. It is spread by droplets from the nose or by contact with fluid from skin blisters. A blistering, itchy rash is usually the most problematic aspect of chickenpox, although occasionally more serious complications can develop.

What to look for ...

1 A mild fever, slightly raised temperature or tiredness.

2 Small, itchy, dark-red spots, which appear in crops, usually starting with the trunk and face and spreading over the rest of the body, including the scalp and genital area. Tiny blisters may also appear in the mouth. Some children have a few spots, others hundreds.

3 Fluid-filled blisters, which develop from the spots and then crust over to form scabs.

What to do ...

1 Keep your child cool and well hydrated.

2 For a fever, give your child a medication such as acetaminophen or ibuprofen. Never give aspirin as there is a possible risk that Reye's syndrome (a rare illness affecting the brain and liver) can be caused by giving aspirin to children suffering from viral infections, especially chickenpox.

3 Encourage your child not to scratch. To relieve itching, apply calamine lotion, a bicarbonate of soda paste, lavender oil or a cold compress, or put your child in a cool bath with oatmeal and baking soda added.

★ Occasionally, serious complications such as encephalitis, arthritis, meningitis (see p.43) or bronchopneumonia can develop. CALL YOUR DOCTOR if your child seems seriously ill, has a temperature above 103°F (39.4°C) or if the rash becomes infected.

Take note ...

✎ Chickenpox can be life-threatening for children who have a disease that affects the immune system, such as leukemia or AIDS.

✎ A vaccine is available, and is usually effective at preventing the disease (see p.15).

✎ IF A PREGNANT WOMAN catches chickenpox, especially in the first three months of pregnancy or before delivery, THE FETUS OR NEWBORN BABY MAY BE INFECTED. This can result in problems such as growth retardation, brain damage, scarring, malformations and cataracts. If you are pregnant and have been in contact with the virus, your immunity should be checked.

✎ The chickenpox virus may reactivate years later, and cause shingles (see p.48).

shingles

variable

CONTAGIOUS—
CAN CAUSE
CHICKENPOX

UNCOMMON
IN CHILDREN

INCUBATION PERIOD

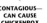

➡ Also called herpes zoster, shingles is a reactivation of the chickenpox virus (varicella-zoster), which lies dormant in a spinal or cranial nerve root after someone has had chickenpox (see p.47). It is uncommon in children, especially those under the age of 10, and is usually mild.

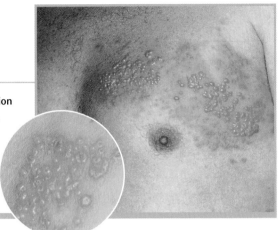

What to look for ...

1 Tingling, tenderness or prickling pain a few days before a rash develops.

2 A one-sided, red rash with papules (tiny red spots), which evolve into vesicles (fluid-filled blisters). These are similar to those occurring in chickenpox. The vesicles appear along the skin path supplied by a particular nerve — usually in the trunk. Medically, this is known as a dermatome pattern — a dermatome is an area of skin served by a single spinal nerve. The rash may be painful and itchy. The vesicles become pustular and crust over before healing within two to three weeks.

★ Depressed white scars may be left when the vesicles heal.

★ Shingles cannot occur in someone who has not already had chickenpox.

What to do ...

1 CALL YOUR DOCTOR. Specific treatment is not usually necessary for children with shingles, but your doctor may prescribe an analgesic for any pain and advise rest. Oral antiviral drugs are not normally recommended for children, but acyclovir may be prescribed.

2 Keep your child away from persons who have not had chickenpox; the virus shed from shingles can cause chickenpox in a nonimmune person.

★ If the area around the eye is involved (ophthalmic shingles), urgent referral to an ophthalmologist (eye specialist) is required.

★ If bacterial infection of the vesicles occurs, a topical antibacterial medication is needed.

Take note ...

✎ There is no link between the severity of the rash and the severity of the pain.

✎ The most common complication is secondary bacterial infection of the vesicles.

✎ Children who have shingles and a generalized chickenpoxlike rash may have a serious underlying illness such as leukemia.

hand, foot & mouth disease

FAIRLY COMMON

4–6 days

INCUBATION PERIOD

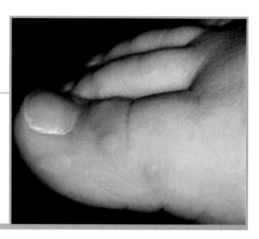

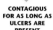

➡ This mild infection, which can occur either in epidemics or more sporadically, has nothing to do with the foot and mouth disease suffered by cattle. The disease is caused by the virus Coxsackie A16, or occasionally by other viruses of the same group, and is most common in young children.

What to look for ...

1 Tiny mouth ulcers or blisters, which appear on the lips, tongue, gums and the inside of the cheeks.

2 Small, round or oval, reddish papules, progressing to grayish blisters surrounded by redness, which appear one or two days later on the palms, hands, forearms and the soles of the feet. Sometimes, the blisters spread to other sites such as the armpits or buttocks.

3 Slight fever, headache or malaise.

4 Mild difficulty in swallowing and a reluctance to eat.

What to do ...

1 To help relieve any discomfort, give your child a soothing mouthwash (ask your pharmacist to recommend one suitable for your child), or a nonaspirin medication such as acetaminophen or ibuprofen.

2 Avoid giving your child fruit juice as this can irritate the mouth ulcers.

★ Although there is no way to treat the disease itself, it will usually clear spontaneously in about seven days.

Take note ...

✎ Hand washing is important in the prevention of coxsackie viruses, especially after going to the toilet.

✎ Although both conditions are caused by the Coxsackie virus, hand, foot and mouth disease should not be confused with herpangina, an infection of the throat with very similar symptoms, but no skin lesions. Herpangina usually clears in about seven days, and can be treated in the same way as hand, foot and mouth disease.

✎ The skin lesions disappear within a few days, but the mouth ulcers may take more than a week to disappear.

roseola infantum

5–15 days

CONTAGIOUS
UNTIL RASH
DISAPPEARS

COMMON IN
CHILDREN

INCUBATION PERIOD

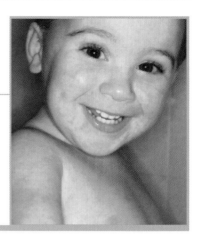

➜ Also called exanthem subitum, or sixth disease, this is a viral
illness caused by the human herpes virus 6 (HHV-6) — a different type
of herpes virus to those that cause cold sores. It is characterized by
the sudden onset of a high fever and a rash, which appears as the
fever ends. There is a very small risk of a febrile convulsion (a fit
caused by high temperature).

What to look for ...

1 Fever and a high temperature of around
103–105°F (39.5–40.5°C), which lasts for
about four days before returning to normal.
2 A widespread, red-pink rash, which
appears as the fever ends, with flat spots that
blanch (turn white) when you touch them.
The roseola rash begins on the chest,
stomach, back and neck, and may spread to
the face, arms and legs. It usually lasts for
24 to 48 hours.
★ Your child may also have swollen glands
or be irritable, but should otherwise be well.

What to do ...

1 Reduce your child's temperature. This is
important in order to avoid the possibility of
a febrile convulsion (a fit caused by a high
temperature). Keep your child cool and give
him or her plenty of fluids. Tepid sponging
may help to reduce the fever.

2 Your doctor may advise giving your child a
nonaspirin medication such as acetaminophen
or ibuprofen to reduce the high temperature.
Antibiotics are not effective for treating viral
illnesses like roseola infantum.

Take note ...

✎ The infection usually affects children
between 6 months and 3 years.
✎ Since the diagnosis may be unclear until
the roseola rash appears, your doctor may
order tests such as a blood or urine test to
make sure there is no other infection causing
your child's fever.
✎ One attack provides a child with lasting
immunity (protection against another attack
of the disease).

cold sores (herpes simplex)

2–14 days

CONTAGIOUS—
MAY REMAIN IN
SALIVA FOR
SEVERAL WEEKS

VERY
COMMON

INCUBATION PERIOD

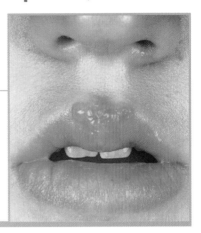

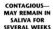 Cold sores are caused by the herpes simplex virus. They usually appear on the lip, around the mouth or nose, or, more rarely, around the eyes or genitals. Most people are exposed to the virus when young. The infection is caught through sharing infected towels and washcloths or through direct skin contact with a cold sore such as may occur when kissing.

What to look for ...

1 Burning, tingling and itching skin may occur before the sore appears.

2 Reddened skin and a raised blotch, or several blotches, which swell and form fluid-filled blisters either singly or in clusters. The blisters form a weeping sore with clear fluid oozing out.

3 A crusty scab that forms as the fluid dries and under which healing takes place.

What to do ...

1 Apply treatment at the first sign of a cold sore. Products which can be bought from pharmacists include antivirals such as acyclovir cream, povidone-iodine paint and

THE **NATURAL** APPROACH

Traditional remedies include cold tea or coffee, ice, lemon juice, lavender oil, half a clove of garlic and witch hazel. To treat the sores, apply one of these remedies several times a day.

antiseptic lotions, creams and gels. Although these will not prevent a recurrence of the virus, they can help reduce discomfort and quicken the healing process a little.

2 Always wash your hands after applying medication.

3 Encourage your child not to touch or pick at the cold sore.

Take note ...

✎ After the first infection the virus remains dormant in the nervous tissue, where triggers such as strong sunlight, colds or stress may cause it to be reactivated.

✎ People with cold sores should avoid kissing other people. In particular, never let anyone with a cold sore kiss a child who has eczema. This can result in a life-threatening infection known as eczema herpeticum.

✎ Young babies and immuno-suppressed children can become dangerously ill if they pick up the herpes virus and this spreads. CALL YOUR DOCTOR if you think your child is at risk.

warts

CONTAGIOUS WHILE WARTS REMAIN

VERY COMMON

months

INCUBATION PERIOD

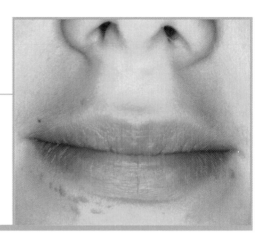

➔ Caused by the human papilloma virus, warts are harmless, painless lumps on the skin, which can adopt a variety of shapes and sizes. Warts are very common in children and can affect any part of the body, but most commonly appear on the hands and feet. Warts on the feet are called verrucae or plantar warts (see p.53).

What to look for ...

common warts

Small, rough, flesh-colored growths, which may grow larger with a grayish cauliflower-like surface. They may be single or multiple, and several may join together. The warts often affect the hands and are most common in children aged between 5 and 10.

plane warts

Small, flat-topped, pink, brown or flesh-colored lumps, with a smooth, slightly raised surface. In children, they usually occur on the face and hands. Plane warts may be multiple and tend to persist for years.

filiform warts

Long, threadlike warts, usually found on your child's face.

genital warts

Soft, fleshy warts around the genital areas. These may be transmitted from elsewhere on the body or may be sexually transmitted.

What to do ...

★ Warts may disappear without treatment, but may take months or years to do so. If you do wish to treat them, try the following:

1 Treat the warts with one of the topical preparations available, such as gels or paint containing salicylic acid, lactic acid or formaldehyde. These cause the layers of flat, dead cells on the skin surface to peel off. Irritation may occur, and the surrounding skin should be protected with petroleum jelly. Do not apply to the face or broken skin.

2 If these treatments are not successful, ask your doctor for advice on using laser surgery, cryotherapy, cautery or curettage (see p.82).

★ See box, right, for advice on natural remedies for warts and verrucae.

Take note ...

✎ Warts are passed by direct contact with an infected person when the virus enters damaged skin through cuts or scratches.

✎ Children who are immuno-compromised or who have atopic eczema are especially susceptible to warts.

verrucae

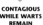

CONTAGIOUS WHILE WARTS REMAIN

COMMON IN CHILDREN

months

INCUBATION PERIOD

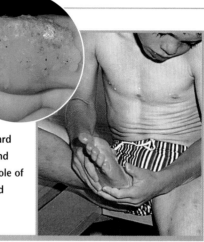

➡ Also called plantar warts, verrucae are common warts (see p.52) that have been caused by body weight pressure to grow inward and penetrate deeply under the skin. They mainly affect children and young adults and usually occur on the weight-bearing part of the sole of the foot — the ball and heel. The virus is usually caught by the child walking barefooted in communal areas such as changing rooms.

What to look for ...

1 Dark-brownish, rough, crumbly lesions, speckled with black dots, appearing singly or in multiples.

2 Plaquelike lesions (known as mosaic warts) made up of multiple, small, tightly packed, individual warts.

3 Pain caused when walking, due to pressure, overlying hard skin, infection or inflammation of the wart.

What to do ...

★ Verrucae may disappear spontaneously, but treatment may be needed if they are painful. If you do wish to treat the verruca, consider trying one of the following:

1 Treat the verruca with one of the topical preparations available from the pharmacist. These include products called keratolytics, which may contain salicylic acid, lactic acid or formaldehyde. The verruca may take a few weeks to completely disappear.

2 Use a pumice stone or emery board to pare away overlying hard skin, and apply a salicylic acid pad.

3 Soak the verruca in a solution of formalin once daily for 10 to 15 minutes, and then rub down the hard skin. This treatment is best for mosaic verrucae.

4 If none of these treatments are successful, ask your doctor about others such as cautery, cryotherapy or laser surgery (see p.82).

★ Cover the warts with a verruca sock or waterproof tape when your child goes swimming, to prevent their transmission.

Take note ...

✎ A verruca can sometimes be confused with a callus (hard skin).

THE **NATURAL** APPROACH

Traditional folklore remedies designed to "charm" away warts and verrucae are numerous, although most are of questionable benefit. Effective treatments include rubbing the warts with a crushed garlic clove or garlic juice, and applying lemon juice, tea tree oil or the juice from dandelion stalks.

molluscum contagiosum

  wks/months

CONTAGIOUS
WHILE WARTS
REMAIN

COMMON IN
CHILDREN

INCUBATION PERIOD

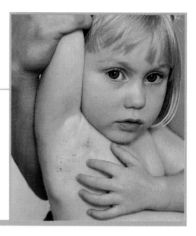

➔ Sometimes called "water warts," this infection is caused by a virus belonging to the poxvirus family. The infection is most common in children under 5 and is spread on the skin by "autoinoculation" — by touching or scratching a lesion and transferring the virus to a new area of skin. It may be spread to others by close physical contact, or by indirect contact such as sharing towels.

What to look for ...

Pearly white, donut-shaped bumps about $\frac{1}{16}$–$\frac{2}{16}$ in (2–5 mm) in diameter. The smooth, firm bumps tend to appear in crops and may have a sunken center ("umbilicated") containing a plug of white, waxy material. The wartlike lesions can appear anywhere on your child's body, including the buttocks and genital area. They are not painful or tender, but may itch.

What to do ...

★ No treatment is usually necessary and the lesions will often simply disappear after several months.
★ The "warts" may sometimes be treated for cosmetic reasons or to prevent the infection spreading. The aim of the treatment is to remove the soft center, after which the bump should go away without undue discomfort or scarring.
★ The doctor may puncture the bumps and touch the center with a sharpened wooden "orange stick" dipped in phenol. Other treatments include: cryosurgery, where the individual bumps are frozen with liquid nitrogen; curettage, where the doctor scrapes the bumps with a sharp, spoon-shaped instrument to remove the centers; and topical therapy, where the bumps are treated with products containing salicylic acid, cantharidin or an antiseptic paint containing providoneiodine.

Take note ...

✎ Children with eczema may be more susceptible to molluscum contagiosum.
✎ Genital area involvement is more common in adults; in children, it may be a sign of sexual abuse.
✎ The lesions may remain unchanged for six to nine months or longer and then disappear spontaneously.
✎ Secondary infection can cause complications.

4 Insect bites & infestations

Your child will inevitably be the recipient of numerous bites and stings while he or she is growing up. Taking proper precautions can help to limit these, of course, but bites remain a common childhood occurrence. In some areas insects can spread disease — some ticks, for example, can cause Lyme disease — and very rarely a bite or sting can provoke a severe allergic reaction, which may even be life threatening. Also, severe itching may result in broken skin from your child's scratching, which can then lead to infection.

However, most insect bites or stings, although they can be painful or irritating, provoke only a mild reaction. Marks on the skin will usually disappear by the next day and do not require medical treatment.

Infestations are another matter. Here, your child will become host to a number of insect parasites, living on the skin or in his or her immediate environment, which will continue to torment your child until banished. Although infestations do not usually cause serious physical harm, they frequently provoke anxiety, horror or shame. Infestations are common, however, and are not caused by poor hygiene. They are also easily treated, although some, such as head lice, often recur in young children.

insect bites & stings

Ants, mosquitoes and flies

Bites or stings from these insects usually result in little more than a localized stinging or burning sensation, swelling, itching and a red bump or spot. In most cases, the itching will disappear in a few hours to a few days. The extent of the reaction will depend on your child's sensitivity — the anticlotting compounds in a mosquito's saliva, for example, cause most children only a mild swelling and itching, but occasionally can result in intense irritation.

Fire ants, which are found throughout the southern United States, can be a particularly painful and distressing pest, since children who disturb a nest are likely to be stung several times, each sting causing a sharp burning sensation and an itchy blister. However, even a fire ant sting will not usually cause your child any serious harm, although — very rarely — a serious allergic reaction may occur (see box, p.57).

Treatment

Apply a cold compress or ice to the area where your child has been bitten or stung to relieve any immediate pain. You may also wish to apply one of the topical products available for the treatment of bites or stings, such as calamine lotion or cream, sprays or creams containing local anesthetic, or witch hazel gel or sticks. Check with your pharmacist that the medications are suitable for children. Other products available to treat stings and bites include devices that release a harmless electric current when clicked over the bite, which may help to dissipate swelling and reduce itching, and small vacuum pumps that draw out irritants using suction. Encourage your child not to scratch the bite as this may make the soreness worse or lead to infection. If the itching is severe, hydrocortisone ointment or oral antihistamines may be needed.

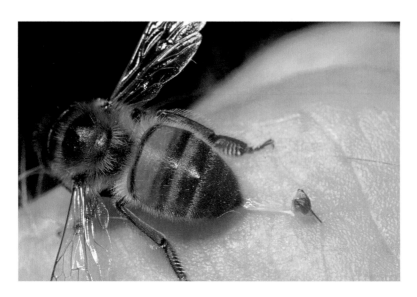

Children often find bites and stings from insects such as bees or mosquitoes painful and irritating, but they are rarely dangerous.

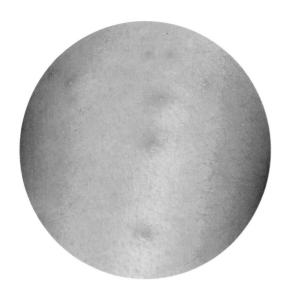

Although the mosquito's thin, sharp proboscis is usually too narrow to stimulate nerve receptors, your child will soon be aware of the itching, swelling and redness caused by the body's allergic reaction to the bite.

Repellents

Always use an insect repellent that is suitable for children, such as those containing natural substances such as aloe vera, lemon, eucalyptus or citronella, and reapply as directed. Products containing DEET should not be used on children under the age of 4 and after that age used sparingly, since it is absorbed through the skin and is potentially harmful. The American Academy of Pediatrics (AAP) advises that products used on children should contain no more than 10 percent DEET. In countries where malaria is a problem, a mosquito bite can be fatal, so putting screens on windows, an insect net over your child's bed and ensuring he or she takes an antimalarial prophylaxis as advised by the doctor, are all essential precautions.

Wasps and bees

If an insect such as a wasp or bee stings your child, its venom is injected into the skin, causing pain and a red mark at the site of the sting. If you can see the stinger — a tiny black dot or small hard point on the mark — do not squeeze it, as you may release more venom. Instead, gently scrape it with a flat knife, your fingernail or a plastic credit card. Do not use tweezers as the sting may break off. Small vacuum pumps, designed for this purpose, can be used to draw out the venom.

Applying a cold compress or ice will help to relieve any immediate pain. Other remedies include anti-sting cream, meat tenderizer (one part tenderizer to five parts water) or essential oils such as lavender or camomile (see p.86). Bicarbonate of soda is an effective way to reduce the pain from bee stings, while vinegar is a useful remedy for wasp stings. In most cases the symptoms are mild but, rarely, severe life-threatening reactions can occur (see box, below).

HEALTH **ALERT** ...

ANAPHYLACTIC SHOCK

Seek medical help immediately if your child has sudden difficulty in breathing, generalized swelling, hives or itching all over the body, or if he or she collapses or falls unconscious. In a small proportion of the population, stings from insects such as bees or fire ants can cause a serious — sometimes fatal — reaction known as anaphylactic shock. You should also get immediate medical attention if your child is stung in the mouth, as there is a risk that the swelling may obstruct his or her airways. If your child has suffered a severe reaction from insect stings in the past, your doctor may advise carrying a prefilled syringe of epinephrine (adrenaline) to use in the event of an emergency.

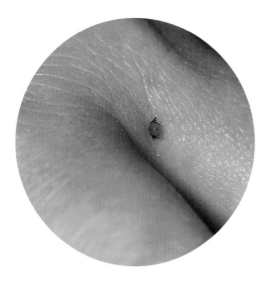

Preventing bites and stings

Encourage your child to wear long-sleeved clothing and long pants if you know he or she will be exposed to insects, especially at dusk. Avoid clothing with bright colors or flowery prints, and don't let your child use scented soap or perfumes, as these are attractive to insects.

Stagnant water is a breeding ground for mosquitoes, so avoid visiting ponds, especially after dark. Many insects are attracted to garbage and to uncovered food, and are often found in orchards or near flowers in bloom. Help prevent

Children sometimes pick up ticks while walking through long grass or other vegetation, particularly when areas of skin, such as the legs, are exposed.

stings by covering up food — especially sweet, sugary foods — and ensuring that your child wears shoes around fallen fruit.

Ticks

These tiny, spiderlike, parasitic creatures attach themselves to the skin of warm-blooded animals — including humans — by their mouths, living off their host's blood. Ticks are not usually painful, although your child may well find the presence of these uninvited hitchhikers extremely distressing. Very rarely, however, ticks may carry a type of bacteria in their stomachs that can cause Lyme disease (see p.32), and so they should be carefully removed.

Removing ticks

Do not use chemicals on the tick or attempt to burn it. Grasp the tick firmly with fine pointed tweezers, as close to the skin surface as possible and pull straight back with a slow, steady force. Avoid crushing the tick's body. Wash the area well with soap and water. If the head stays in your child's skin when the tick is removed, the wound may become infected. Contact your doctor if there is any sign of infection.

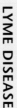

infestations

Lice

Lice are blood-sucking, wingless insects that are transmitted by close contact with an infected person. An infestation of lice is known as pediculosis, since the three species of lice that infest humans come from the *Pediculus* genus. Of these three species, body lice are rare and do not usually affect children. However, head lice are common in school-age children, and pubic lice occasionally can be found in children's eyebrows and eyelashes. The return of children to schools and playgroups after the summer break usually results in a rise in infestations.

Head lice

The head louse, known medically as *Pediculus capitis*, infests only the head hair. Anyone can catch head lice but they are most common in 4- to 11-year-olds and occur in girls more than boys. Head lice do not hop, jump or fly: nearly all infestations result from direct head-to-head contact, although they can also be passed on by

Often, the only symptom that your child has an infestation of head lice will be itching, but this may not start until weeks or months after the infection. It is therefore worthwhile keeping an eye on your child's hair for other indications that he or she has pediculosis. It may be possible to see louse droppings as black specks (similar to pepper) on pillows or collars. Your child may also have a rash on the back of the neck caused by an allergic reaction to louse feces. Another indicator of lice infestation is the presence of tear-shaped eggs or empty eggshells (nits), found further down the hair shaft. The only reliable method of confirming an infection, however, is by finding a live louse. These can be difficult to see with the naked eye and usually are identified while wet combing (see p.60).

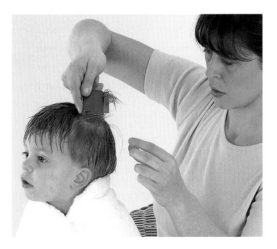

sharing personal belongings such as hats or towels. Lice are found on both dirty and clean, and long and short hair. In most cases of infection, fewer than ten lice are on the head. The female louse lays about six to eight eggs a day, and the eggs take seven to ten days to hatch, leaving the eggshell or "nit" attached to the hair.

Combing, using a special lice detector comb, is an effective way to check your child's hair for evidence of a lice infestation.

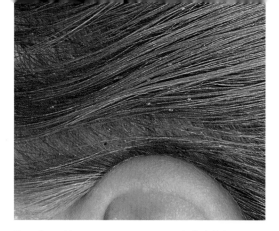

Tear-shaped louse eggs or empty eggshells (nits) can often be seen glued to the hair near the scalp, and may be mistaken for dandruff.

Wet combing

This is one of the most effective ways of detecting a lice infestation, and can also be used to remove lice without the need for insecticides. Wash your child's hair in the normal way, and apply lots of hair conditioner. Comb with an ordinary comb and then — using a fine, lice-detector comb — slowly comb from the roots of the hair through to the tips. Work your way around your child's head and check the teeth of the comb after each stroke, wiping it with a tissue. If any lice are found, repeat the procedure every three to four days for two weeks (to ensure that you remove any newly hatched lice). Alternatively, if you do find lice using the wet comb, you may prefer to use an insecticide to remove them from your child's hair.

Insecticides

These contain malathion, phenothrin, permethrin or carbaryl. Products containing malathion or carbaryl should not be used more than once a week for three weeks at a time, and carbaryl treatments can only be obtained on prescription from your doctor. Check also with your doctor if your child is under 6 months or suffers from asthma or eczema, since the lice preparations can irritate sensitive skin. Follow the instructions on the product carefully. If live lice can still be seen, or are still present within a day or two of treatment, they may be resistant to the insecticide. In this case, use the wet combing method or switch to a product with a different ingredient. The eggs take seven to ten days to hatch, so a second application is recommended after this period has elapsed. Treatment should only be used when head lice have been detected and never to prevent the lice.

Other treatments

To prevent reinfection, wash all your child's bed clothes and clothing on a hot cycle, wash combs and brushes with hot water and soap, and vacuum floors and furniture. Other family members may be infected, and if the presence of lice is confirmed, also will need to be treated. You should also inform your child's school.

No reliable evidence has been published to show that methods such as a battery-operated comb, herbal remedies, tea tree oil or other essential oils are effective in treating head lice. Some essential oils irritate the skin and may not be suitable for children, so use these cautiously, if at all, and not as a preventive measure.

Pubic (crab) lice

This species of louse affects body hair, and only very rarely the hair on the head. Pubic lice are most likely to be found on a child's eyebrows or eyelashes. Watch out for scratching and irritation, with yellow crusting along the edge of the eyelashes. Head lice formulations in aqueous form can be used to remove pubic lice; you may want to ask your doctor to remove any lice from the eyelashes. Alternatively, use petroleum jelly, smoothed on the eyebrows and eyelashes twice a day for ten days, to kill the lice as they hatch.

Scabies

This highly irritating, infectious skin infestation is caused by a mite called *Sarcoptes scabiei* burrowing through the upper layers of the skin. The mites cause an allergic reaction, resulting in an intense itch that often gets worse at night, and an eczema-type rash with papules or nodules and short scaly lesions. Sores or scabs may appear on your child's wrists, between the fingers and toe spaces, in the armpits and on the elbows, chest or genitalia. In infants, the head, neck, palms and soles of the feet also may be affected. There also may be burrow marks, and marks on the skin where the child has been scratching. Scabies is caught by close physical contact between people, such as holding hands, and outbreaks may occur where there is close proximity between children, such as in nurseries. Other family members and close contacts are often similarly affected. Scabies may be infectious for two to four weeks before itching starts.

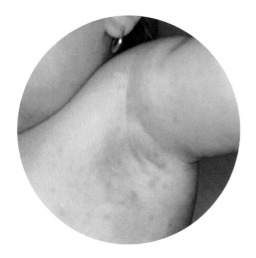

The scabies mite prefers warm, protected skin folds and crevices such as the armpits or the spaces between the fingers and toes.

Treatment

If you think that your child may have scabies, call your doctor, who may wish to do a test involving skin scraping in order to make the diagnosis. There are a variety of creams and lotions to treat scabies, such as those containing malathion or permethrin; your doctor will prescribe a suitable one. All household members should be treated at the same time. Your child will be clear of infection 24 hours after treatment, but a second application is usually recommended four days later. The lesions may remain and cause itching for several weeks, so an anti-itch cream such as calamine lotion or antihistamine tablets may also be needed. Although there is usually little risk of transferring the infestation via clothing or skin scales, such transfer is possible with crusted scabies — a less common type of scabies characterized by a heavy infestation — and clothing and bed linen should be laundered.

APPLYING THE **SCABICIDE** ...

The lotion or cream should be applied to the entire skin surface from the neck down, paying particular attention to the webs of the fingers and toes. Remember also to treat under the fingernails and reapply if the hands are washed. If your infant is affected, the cream or lotion should also be applied to the scalp, neck and face. Babies and young children should wear mittens to prevent them sucking off the scabicide. A hot bath is not necessary before applying the treatment and may increase the absorption of the scabicide into the bloodstream, removing it from the skin.

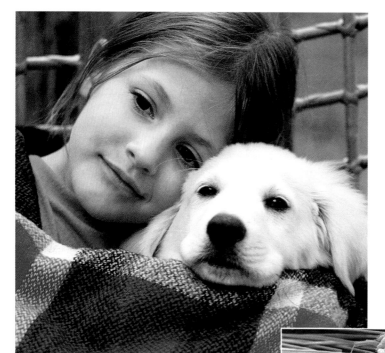

Many common species of flea prefer to feed on animals rather than humans. Although households with pets often have infestations, the fleas will usually bite the pet owners only when they are unable to feed on the cat or dog. In contrast, humans are the preferred host of the common bedbug (*below*).

Fleas

Fleas are most likely to be a problem in homes that have domestic pets such as cats and dogs. Look for crops of small, itchy, red bumps, which are often in groups in areas where there is close contact with clothing, such as around the waist. The itching from the bites will vary according to your child's sensitivity. It may also be possible to see the fleas themselves in pet fur, or on carpets or furniture; they are excellent jumpers and can leap several inches when disturbed.

Irritation from the bites can be relieved by a topical application of calamine lotion or 1 percent hydrocortisone cream, and oral antihistamines, if necessary. You should also vacuum regularly, treat your pet and soft furnishings, and spray your garden. A vet can give advice on which insecticides are best to use.

Bedbugs

Bedbugs often live in nooks and crannies around the room or on furniture, as well as in the bedding itself. They bite at night and may be difficult to spot. Bedbug bites look like groups of itchy red spots surrounded by a blister, and are usually found on exposed skin such as on the hands and face. Relieve the itching, if necessary, with a topical application of calamine lotion or 1 percent hydrocortisone cream, or with oral antihistamines. You also should contact your state pesticide agency or a pest control specialist for help to clear a house infestation.

Lumps, bumps & bruises

Most children have minor accidents as they grow up. Few of these accidents are serious, but they often result in minor cuts and grazes, burns or bruises. Other swellings or lumps in your child's skin, such as boils or whitlows, occur as a result of bacterial or viral infections. While these are often painful, they, too, are rarely serious. They are not normally infectious, and your child is not usually ill.

It is important, however, to keep a close eye on all of these lumps, bumps and bruises. If large or recurrent bruises appear without any apparent reason or in areas where bruises would not normally appear, such as the abdomen, always have them checked with your doctor to eliminate any serious disorders. Similarly, if your child has repeated boils, or a painful or infected swelling of the skin, you should contact your doctor for advice. Larger swellings of the glands may mean your child has caught an infectious disease such as glandular fever or mumps. Always contact your doctor if your child has swollen glands or an unexplained swelling in any other part of the body.

lumps, bumps & bruises

Blisters

When fluid (serum) collects between the two layers of the skin, the dermis and epidermis, it causes a fluid-filled swelling or bubble, which may feel hot, itchy or painful. Blisters may occur as a result of severe sunburn, an insect bite or allergy, a burn or as part of an infectious rash. Rarely, blistering of your child's skin may be the result of a genetic disorder. The most common cause of blisters is friction, such as when a new shoe rubs the heel of your child's foot.

Treatment

Most blisters are sterile and will heal naturally, but a burst blister may become infected. If the blister breaks, or if further irritation or injury is likely, cover the area with a blister pad, adhesive bandage or a clean, dry dressing, and a dab of antiseptic cream. If your child has large or multiple blisters, such as those caused by sunburn, scalding or allergies, or if your child develops blisters for no obvious reason, you should have them checked by a doctor.

Bruises

Most children acquire bruises from time to time, in the course of everyday play or as a result of accidental injury. A knock or blunt blow to the skin can cause the leakage of blood from capillaries into the surrounding tissues, resulting in a discolored area of skin, which may also be painful and swollen. The bruises may appear hours or days after an injury. Most bruises will disappear by themselves within a few days to a couple of weeks, but holding a cold compress or ice pack to the area will help reduce pain and swelling. See your doctor if the bruising is extensive or unexplained: it may be caused by underlying injuries such as fractures, by hematological (blood) disorders, or may even be the result of abuse. Occasionally, young children may have what appear to be bruises on the buttocks or back, but which are actually Mongolian spots, a harmless birthmark (see p.72).

Never burst a blister. The fluid inside blisters is usually sterile and will eventually be reabsorbed, but if burst it may become infected.

Boils and carbuncles

A boil occurs when an infection develops at the root of a hair follicle, under the skin. The cause of the infection is usually the staphylococcus bacteria. Boils are most common in hairy or damp places such as the armpits or groin. They may also occur where there is rubbing, such as underneath a collar. Look for a warm and tender red lump, which may throb painfully. Over the next two to three days the boil swells with pus and becomes more painful. As it gets bigger, a yellowish head or center develops, which eventually bursts through the skin. Once the pus escapes, the pain is relieved. If the boil has multiple heads or if several boils join together, this is called a carbuncle.

Children who are at particular risk of getting boils include those who suffer from diabetes mellitus or anemia, or children who have an immunodeficiency disease such as leukemia. If your child has large or recurring boils, your doctor may wish to perform a blood test to check for undiagnosed conditions.

Treatment

Do not squeeze the boil. Apply a hot compress several times a day to relieve the pain and hasten the bursting of the boil. If your child has a particularly unsightly or painful boil, you may wish to see your doctor. If the boil is ready to burst, the doctor may make a small cut in the center to help the pus to drain, and may also prescribe antibiotics to kill the bacteria. You should always see your doctor if your child has a carbuncle, since surgical drainage or antibiotics may be needed.

Cysts

These are normally harmless swellings of various sizes, filled with fluid or semisolid matter. See acne (p.35) and milia (p.20).

Chilblains

Known medically as perniosis, chilblains are raised, round, shiny, purple-red swellings on the fingers or toes, which may be itchy or even painful. Chilblains are caused by excessive narrowing of small blood vessels below the skin, as a reaction to a cold environment. They are less common today — a result of central heating. To prevent chilblains, make sure your child wears well-insulated gloves and footwear. Chilblains

The swelling and itching of chilblains can be avoided by ensuring all parts of your child's body, especially the hands and feet, are kept warm and dry in cold weather.

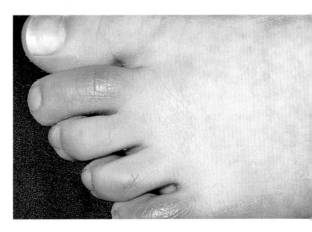

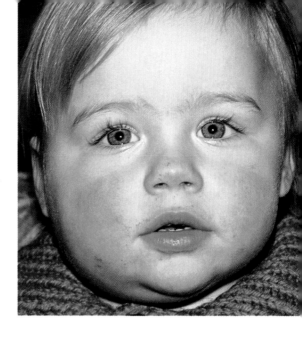

The most common symptom of mumps is a swelling of the salivary glands near the ears. This swelling can occur on one or both sides of your child's head.

generally heal without treatment, but chilblain or arnica cream helps to control your child's itching and promote healing.

Glandular fever

Also known as infectious mononucleosis, glandular fever is a common viral infection caused by a herpes virus known as the Epstein-Barr virus. It is characterized by rubbery swellings — swollen glands — which can be felt under the skin on the neck, armpits and throat. Your child may also suffer from tiredness, fever, headache and a sore throat. Sometimes there may be jaundice, difficulty in breathing, chest pain and a widespread pink rash. The disease, which has an incubation period of around four to seven weeks, is transmitted by contact with saliva — hence its nickname "the kissing disease."

Treatment

If you think that your child may have glandular fever, you should contact your doctor, who will confirm the diagnosis with a blood test. There is

HEALTH **ALERT** ...

If your child is suffering from glandular fever, you should call your doctor immediately if he or she has sudden abdominal pain or other significant symptoms. On rare occasions, an enlarged spleen may rupture, causing blood loss and shock.

GLANDULAR FEVER

no specific treatment, but your child should have plenty of bed rest, especially if the infection is severe. Normally your child will make a full recovery, but may be tired for several months. In this case strenuous exercise should be avoided.

Mumps

This viral infection, which mainly affects unimmunized children over the age of 2, is spread by direct contact with saliva or airborne droplets. The infection causes a swelling of the parotid salivary glands (the glands that produce saliva) at the back of the cheeks. In most cases, mumps begins with the swelling of one gland in front of the ear and over the jaw. A day or two later, the opposite gland may also swell, although in some cases the swelling is restricted to just the one side. Your child may have pain or earache when chewing or swallowing and be unwell with a headache and fever. Until the 1960s, when the mumps vaccine was first licensed, the disease was very common. Today, all children are offered immunization as part of the measles, mumps and rubella (MMR) program (see p.15).

HEALTH **ALERT** ...

Although it is normally only the parotid glands that are affected, mumps can involve an inflammation of the brain, pancreas or other glands and organs. This can cause complications including viral meningitis, encephalitis, deafness, pancreatitis and — in older males — orchitis (inflammation of the testicles), so it is important to monitor your child's condition and symptoms closely.

Treatment

If your child finds swallowing painful, give him or her plenty of fluids and soft foods. A non-aspirin painkiller such as acetaminophen or ibuprofen can help to bring down any fever and relieve pain. You should also let your doctor know that your child has mumps. Call your doctor immediately, however, if your child seems seriously ill, has a headache with a stiff neck, swollen testicles, abdominal pain or persistent earache, since these symptoms may indicate serious complications.

Paronychia

This noncontagious infection, uncommon in children, is caused by the inflammation of the folds of skin surrounding the fingernails, and can be acute or chronic. Acute paronychia, which usually lasts only a few days, is most commonly caused by a bacterial infection such as staphylococcus, following injury to the skin around the nail. Fungal (yeast) infections can also be a cause. Chronic paronychia occurs when the cuticle separates and loses its waterproof properties, allowing infection, usually *Candida albicans*, to enter the nail. This causes swelling and further separation of the cuticle and may result in ridging, thickening, discoloration and nail loss. Several nails may be affected. Children who suck their thumbs can develop chronic paronychia, while children with diabetes are also at risk. Sometimes the swelling and infection from a paronychia will increase, and an abscess, called a whitlow or felon, may develop in the fleshy part the finger (see below).

Treatment

If your child has paronychia, you should see your doctor: antifungal or antibiotic drugs may be prescribed, depending on the type of infection. If there is pus, the paronychia may need to be incised. Keep your child's hands as dry as possible and try to avoid frequent contact with water. If your child is in any pain, you can give him or her a nonaspirin medication such as acetaminophen or ibuprofen.

Whitlows (felons)

A whitlow is an abscess in the pulp of the fingertip, which may result from an infection such as acute paronychia. Swelling, redness and throbbing pain in the fingertip develop as the accumulation of pus causes pressure upon the surrounding tissues. If your child has a whitlow you should contact your doctor, who may treat the whitlow with antibiotics, or incise and drain the abscess. A whitlow should never be neglected or ignored as your child's finger bone may become infected (osteomyelitis).

Herpetic whitlows

An inflammation of the nail folds may also be a result of an infection by the herpes simplex virus, resulting in a painful, red swelling around the fingernails. The infection can be distinguished from a normal whitlow by the presence of blisters around the nail. Children or infants with oral herpes can spread the herpes virus from their mouths to their fingernails by sucking their thumbs, and in turn the virus may spread to other parts of the body. If you think your child has a herpetic whitlow you should see your doctor. It usually will not be incised because of the risk of spreading infection, but an antiviral drug may be applied. Recurrent attacks sometimes occur.

Scars

Marks are often left on the skin following an injury such as a burn or cut, or a skin lesion such as acne (see p.35). As the wound begins to heal, a red or purple mark may develop on the skin, and this later becomes white and glistening. At first, a new scar may be itchy or painful. Scars are harmless and many gradually fade, becoming pale or disappearing. See your doctor if a scar becomes unsightly or develops into a keloid (see below), since it may be possible to reduce its size or improve its appearance.

Keloids

Overgrowths of dense, fibrous scar tissue — keloids — are more common in people with dark or black skin, the result of a defective healing process in which an excess of collagen (a fibrous protein) is produced after the wound has healed. The scar at first seems to heal normally, but then continues to grow for some period of time, extending beyond the original injury and becoming larger and thicker. The result is an itchy, thick, raised, hard, irregularly shaped, red- or white-colored scar. Keloids are harmless, but may be unsightly. Some non-keloid scars may also continue to thicken, staying red and raised for some months but — unlike keloids — remaining confined to the area of tissue damage. These are called hypertrophic scars, and should be treated in the same way as keloids.

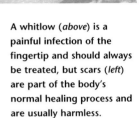

A whitlow (*above*) is a painful infection of the fingertip and should always be treated, but scars (*left*) are part of the body's normal healing process and are usually harmless.

Treatment

If left alone, keloids gradually flatten and fade to become pale and shiny. Early keloids may respond to steroid injections, which may cause shrinkage and reduce irritation. Self-treatment, adhesive, silicone-gel sheets, which are said to flatten, soften and fade new and old scars (up to 20 years old) are available from pharmacies. As these are expensive, and the treatment period is between two and four months, you may wish to discuss their use with your doctor first. Surgical removal of keloids and other scars is usually avoided as a new keloid scar may form.

Skin tags

These are soft, harmless, skin-colored or brown outgrowths of skin, usually found on the neck, groin or anal region. Their precise cause is unknown, although they do seem to run in families. If your child has skin tags that are unsightly or catch on clothing, they can be easily removed by a doctor.

Birthmarks, pigments & growths

About one in every hundred babies has some type of birthmark or what's medically known as a nevus. A birthmark that is present at birth, or shortly after, is known as a congenital nevus, but other nevi, such as freckles or moles, may appear as the child grows older. The marks can appear anywhere on the body and, although they can assume a variety of shapes, colors and sizes, they are all persistent and either discolor the skin or cause it to swell.

Most birthmarks or growths are completely harmless but, in rare cases, a congenital mole or a pigmented patch of skin may sometimes grow and become a malignant melanoma (see p.71). The majority of birthmarks are temporary and eventually disappear without treatment; others may occur on parts of the body where they cannot be seen. However, if your child has a facial birthmark, or a mark somewhere else on the body that is permanent or disfiguring, this may cause your child a lot of embarrassment and distress. Fortunately, a number of treatments are now available that can minimize or completely remove a disfiguring or permanent birthmark, or one that is causing physical problems.

birthmarks, pigments & growths

Pigments and blood vessels

Birthmarks, moles and other nevi develop in children for two reasons. One type, pigmented nevi, occur when there is an incorrect mixture of pigment in the skin. Skin cells, known as melanocytes, produce the pigment, melanin, which is needed to protect the skin from harmful ultraviolet rays. If too much melanin is produced, moles, freckles or other brown patches may develop. The second type, vascular nevi, occur due to abnormalities of the blood vessels. If there are too many blood vessels, red or purple marks may appear on the skin.

Freckles

Many children break out in endearing crops of light-brown freckles every summer, on areas of their body most exposed to the sun. These small, flat patches of pigmented skin usually first appear between the ages of 2 and 4, often becoming darker and larger in sunny weather. The most commonly acquired type of pigmented nevus, freckles often run in families and are most common in children with fair skin. They are not harmful and no treatment is necessary.

Moles

These pigmented spots are made up of melanocytes, the pigment-producing cells, and vary in color from pale brown to black. Moles start out flat, but over time can thicken and become raised with an irregular surface, and may become hairy. When present at birth, moles are known as congenital melanocytic nevi. These congenital moles are more common in fair-skinned people, and tend to grow with the child.

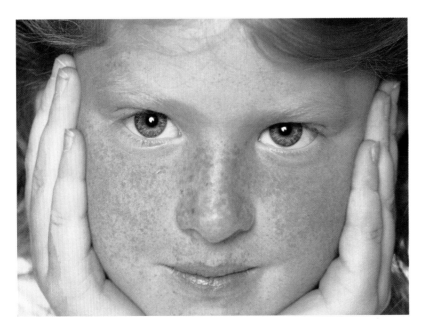

Blond and red-headed children are most prone to freckles. During the summer months, these harmless pigmented spots are most numerous and darkest. They generally fade during the colder, less sunny months.

They are generally larger and deeper than acquired moles, which are not present at birth, but appear during childhood or adolescence.

Treatment

Generally, moles are not removed unless they are unsightly or in an awkward position, in which case they may be surgically removed. Most moles are benign (nonmalignant), but moles that undergo changes will be tested to see if they are cancerous (see box, right). If they are malignant, they will also need to be surgically removed. Congenital moles are more likely to become cancerous than acquired moles, which are seldom a cause for worry. Rarely, a child may be born with an extensive hairy mole, covering a considerable area of skin, usually on the lower torso or buttocks. This type of mole is most predisposed to cancerous changes, so if your child has one, ensure that it is checked regularly.

Melanomas

A comparatively rare, but dangerous form of skin cancer, melanomas develop in the same melanin-producing cells that produce moles. A melanoma usually arises from a congenital or pre-existing mole, but one can occur in areas of previously unblemished skin. Melanomas rarely occur in children under the age of 15, but severe sunburn in childhood can increase the risk, and will certainly increase the likelihood of melanomas occurring later in life. Children who are the most vulnerable are those with blue eyes, fair skin and freckles; children who burn easily in the sun; children who have congenital moles and children with a family history of melanomas.

Treatment

The main preventive measure to take against melanomas consists of avoiding excessive exposure to the sun (see p.12 for advice on

MELANOMAS

HEALTH **ALERT** ...

All moles should be observed regularly for changes. Most pre-existing moles will change as your child grows and the changes are rarely of concern. Use the "ABCD" checklist to help you to remember the major changes to look for in order to spot a melanoma:

A Asymmetry. Most melanomas develop unevenly, and one half of the mole may look different from the other.
B Border. Most melanomas have an irregular or ragged outline.
C Color. Most melanomas have an irregular color, which may vary from a blue-white tinge to a mixture of pink, white, brown, black or intense black. They also may be red, due to inflammation.
D Diameter. Most melanomas are more than ¼ in (6 mm) in diameter. You should also look out for any small brown lesions occuring around the edge of the mole, and any crusting, bleeding, oozing or itching.

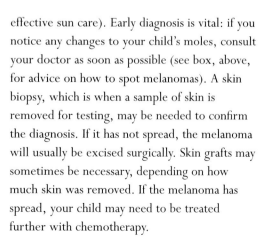

effective sun care). Early diagnosis is vital: if you notice any changes to your child's moles, consult your doctor as soon as possible (see box, above, for advice on how to spot melanomas). A skin biopsy, which is when a sample of skin is removed for testing, may be needed to confirm the diagnosis. If it has not spread, the melanoma will usually be excised surgically. Skin grafts may sometimes be necessary, depending on how much skin was removed. If the melanoma has spread, your child may need to be treated further with chemotherapy.

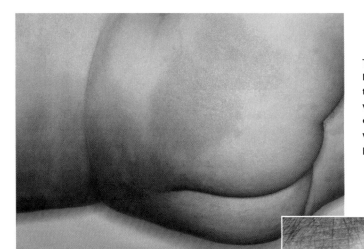

The dark, bruiselike Mongolian spots (*left*) and the irregular white patches of vitiligo (*below*). Both are caused by abnormalities within the child's pigment-producing cells.

Spitz nevus

This fleshy pink-red papule is a rare form of mole, which occurs mainly in children and adolescents. The lesion, which often occurs on the face, can cause parents considerable concern since it may initially grow, resembling a melanoma. It sometimes is called a juvenile melanoma but it is completely benign (non-malignant) and many doctors prefer not to use this name. Spitz nevi are harmless but, because they are so difficult to distinguish from malignant melanomas, they are often removed.

Mongolian spots

These marks, present at birth, are found mainly in black or Asian babies. They are caused by a concentration of the pigment cells (melanocytes) deep in the skin, and usually occur on the buttocks and back, although they sometimes affect the ankles and wrists. Because the large bluish-black marks look so similar to bruises, Mongolian spots sometimes may be misdiagnosed as nonaccidental bruising. However, they do not have any medical significance and will gradually fade as your child gets older.

Vitiligo

Caused by the loss of the pigment melanin, vitiligo is a noninfectious skin disease that can affect any age group, although most cases occur before the age of 20. The pigment loss causes white patches of varying size and shape, looking a little like splashes of spilt milk, which occur most often on the face, backs of hands, armpits and groin. These marks may also continue to spread and change size or shape over time. It is not known why the melanocyte cells stop producing melanin, but it is thought that several factors are involved. These include a genetic link, as vitiligo may run in families. Another theory is that the condition is an autoimmune disorder where the body's immune system reacts against the melanocyte cells and destroys them.

The nonpigmented skin of vitiligo sufferers has little natural protection from the sun and is particularly prone to burning and sun damage. You should ensure your child's skin is well protected from the sun (see p.12 for advice on effective sun care). Vitiligo may occur in conjunction with autoimmune diseases such as diabetes or thyroid disease, so talk to your doctor about having your child tested for these conditions.

Treatment

Vitiligo is not normally a serious health problem, but the patches may be conspicuous or disfiguring — particularly in children with dark skin — and can cause considerable distress. Various treatments can be tried to slow down its progress or improve coloration. Your child may be given topical corticosteroids (see p.80), for a limited period and under the direction of a pediatric dermatologist (a children's skincare specialist). Another option is to try psoralens and ultraviolet light therapy (PUVA). This involves giving your child drugs that make the skin sensitive to light, and then using ultraviolet light to make the color return. You may also wish to use camouflage makeup to disguise the patches.

Café-au-lait patches

These flat, smooth, brown or coffee-colored oval patches are found in around 10 percent of the population and are usually permanent. They are typically small, but may measure an inch or more. Talk to your doctor if your child has several patches, since six or more café-au-lait patches may indicate neurofibromatosis. This is a genetic disorder where soft swellings develop on the nerves of the skin, or elsewhere in the body.

Port-wine stains

Caused by the malformation of the blood capillaries under the skin, port-wine stains are very rare, affecting only around one child in every thousand. Despite this, they are particularly problematic, since they are permanent and disfiguring marks, which grow with the child and do not fade — indeed they may grow darker with age. The bright red or purple stains, which are present at birth, cover a flat, irregular area of skin, usually on the face, neck or head, and are more common in girls than boys. They vary in size and shape, and may become raised and thickened over time. Port-wine stains in visible areas can cause some children considerable psychological problems. Advances in treatment, good family support and a positive attitude can help your child to overcome any difficulties.

Rarely, port-wine stains on the upper eyelid, brow and forehead — which involve a large cranial nerve located in this area called the trigeminal nerve — may be associated with Sturge-Weber syndrome. This is a congenital condition that can cause problems such as epilepsy, mental retardation and visual disturbances. Port-wine stains on the limbs are associated with limb enlargement, a condition known as Klippel-Trenaunay-Weber syndrome.

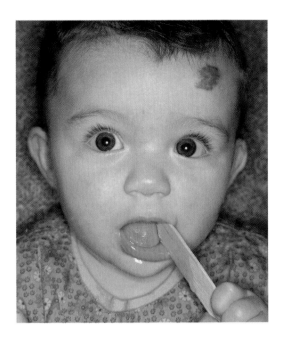

Strawberry marks affect around 1 in every 20 babies, but usually fade over time.

Laser surgery

Camouflage makeup can help to disguise a port-wine stain as the child grows older and more self-conscious, but laser treatment (see p.82) now provides a more permanent option. A pulsed dye laser, the most common type of laser used, is both safe and effective. Laser treatment may not clear the stain completely, but over 80 percent of children with port-wine stains will benefit, with some attaining complete clearance.

Strawberry marks

Known medically as a hemangioma, strawberry marks may also be called strawberry nevi, or capillary hemangioma. They are caused by a proliferation of immature blood capillaries, and consist of a raised red area resembling a strawberry. Strawberry marks are the most common type of hemangioma, but there are other types, including subcutaneous or cavernous hemangiomas, which develop deep under the skin as bluish swellings, and mixed hemangiomas, with both strawberrylike components and bluish swellings. The marks, which develop during the first few weeks of life, are more common in girls and preterm babies. Strawberry nevi are usually found on the head, neck and trunk, and some children may develop several marks.

The majority of strawberry marks disappear, without treatment, by the time your child is seven. They may grow rapidly during the first year of life, but then become static and spontaneously shrink over the next 3 to 4 years. Strawberry hemangiomas may bleed, but severe bleeding is rare. Most bleeding can be dealt with by firm pressure with a dressing or a wad of tissues. Medical treatment should be necessary only if the hemangioma causes problems — if, for example, it is in the mouth and interferes with feeding, if it is near the eye and blocks your child's vision, or if it has a major effect on your child's appearance. Treatments include surgical removal, laser therapy and oral or injected corticosteroids. Very rarely, internal hemangiomas may develop on a site such as the liver, heart or brain and cause serious problems such as heart failure or a blood clotting disorder called Kasabach-Merritt syndrome.

Salmon patches

Also known as stork marks or stork bites, since they often occur on the back of the neck where the mythical stork would have carried a newborn baby, these flat, pink or red patches are also often found on the forehead, the upper eyelids and the root of the nose of newborns. Made up of dilated capillaries, they are harmless, very common and do not need any treatment. A mark on the face normally fades during the first year, although a mark on the neck may remain throughout life.

Treatments

A child's stubborn or unpleasant skin condition should never cause you despair. There are numerous and wide-ranging treatments available, which, in many cases, are extremely effective. Treatments range from complicated surgical techniques at one end of the scale, through to complementary therapies and simple home remedies. The treatment will, to a large extent, depend upon the nature of your child's skin condition.

Most childhood skin problems can be treated in the home, with the use of topical skin preparations applied directly to your child's skin, or with oral medications such as antihistamines or antibiotics, available over the counter or by prescription. Some treatments may produce a permanent cure, others may simply improve the skin condition or keep the problem under control. Sometimes, two or three treatments may be combined, or several tried until a suitable one is found. Other conditions may require a visit to a specialist, who can give more specific advice on how best to treat and protect your child's delicate skin.

If you don't understand how a treatment works, or are worried about any possible side effects, always talk to a health professional.

creams, steroids & other topical skin preparations

The majority of childhood skin problems may be treated simply through the use of topical preparations, such as creams or ointments, applied directly to your child's skin. A vast array of these medications are available, and finding the right medication for your child can be confusing. Many preparations can be bought under both a generic name — the official medical name — and a proprietary or "brand" name chosen by the individual manufacturer. The type of emollient known generically as soft yellow petrolatum, for example, can also be bought under the brand name Vaseline. Check for the product's active ingredients or ask a pharmacist if you are unsure which brand to use.

The cost of skin preparations can vary enormously, but although brand-name products are generally more expensive, they are not necessarily better. A simple aqueous cream is often just as effective for dry skin conditions such as eczema as more expensive proprietary creams.

Types of skin preparation

Medications applied to the skin are usually contained within a preparation known as a base or vehicle. This may simply be used to contain the active ingredients and transport them to the site of treatment, but often is beneficial in itself. To a large extent, the type of vehicle used will depend upon the skin condition your child has.

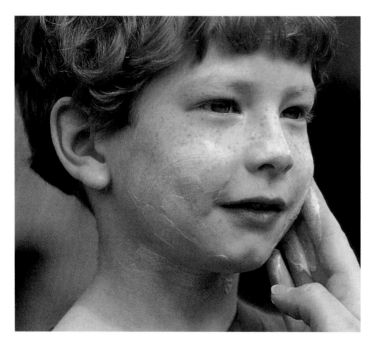

Topical skin preparations are medications, such as creams or lotions, that are applied to your child's skin locally — at the site of the problem. They are the first choice of treatment for a wide range of skin conditions.

Complying with the prescribed treatment is important, especially if your child has an infection, although you should stop medicating immediately if your child has an allergic reaction (see p.22). Always remember that oral medications such as antibiotics should be taken until the course is finished, and topical skin preparations should be applied only as directed. If your child has been prescribed a treatment and you wish to use another preparation, such as a herbal remedy, always inform your doctor first. There may be an adverse reaction, or two different drugs may react with each other.

Creams and ointments

Semisolid, nongreasy emulsions of oil in water, creams may be used on their own for their emollient (moisturizing) properties, or as a vehicle for an ingredient such as hydrocortisone. Because they contain water, and are light and easily absorbed, they are particularly useful for "weepy" or crusted skin. Some creams contain a preservative to prevent the growth of bacteria or fungi, although this may irritate some skins.

Ointments, like creams, can help moisturize the skin. Unlike creams, however, these greasy preparations contain little or no water and are not suitable for use on infected or weeping areas of skin. Ointments are particularly useful for very dry skin, as they impede water loss and seal in moisture. The most commonly used ointment base is soft white petrolatum. When applying creams and ointments to skin lesions such as those caused by impetigo, the skin should not be heavily coated in the belief that more is better. Instead, lightly rub in the prescribed amount of cream or ointment until it is absorbed.

Barrier preparations

These creams and ointments are used to protect the skin against water or irritating substances, such as the ammonia in urine that causes diaper rash. They usually contain water-repellent substances such as dimethicone (a silicone).

Dusting powders and pastes

Made with a base such as talc, starch, kaolin or zinc oxide powder, powders dry the skin and reduce friction by absorbing moisture. They may be used as lubrication in skin folds where friction may occur. Powders may also be used to contain active ingredients such as antifungal drugs or antiseptics, and are often used in the prevention of fungal conditions such as athlete's foot. Powders should be applied lightly and not to very moist areas as they may cake and irritate your child's skin.

Finely powdered solids such as zinc oxide and coal tar may be incorporated into an ointment base to produce a stiff paste, which may be used on its own or impregnated into bandages. Pastes are used to protect the skin and absorb unwanted moisture in conditions where there are skin lesions, such as psoriasis or eczema.

If a young child objects to you applying cream, try making a game of it. Draw a cream face on your child's arm or legs; let him or her look in a mirror when you are applying the cream and tell you when its "all gone"; or let your child apply some cream to a doll at the same time. A baby who is at the kicking or wriggling stage may need distraction, such as an overhead toy to gaze at.

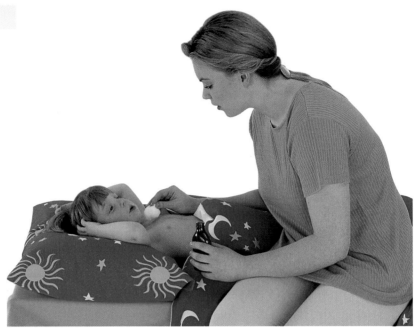

Lotions that have a soothing or cooling effect, such as calamine or witch hazel, can be applied as often as needed. Soak a cotton ball in the solution and gently dab on the skin.

Lotions

These semiliquid preparations are easily applied, especially to large or more hairy areas, and are usually the treatment of choice for conditions such as head lice, scalp psoriasis or scabies. When using lotions to treat conditions such as head lice or scabies you should always ensure that you follow the instructions carefully, since they may irritate the skin.

Shake lotions are suspensions of powder in water (such as calamine lotion) which need to be shaken before use to stop the powder settling on the bottom. When the liquid evaporates, they leave a deposit of fine powder on the skin that encourages scabs to form.

Collodions

Painted on the skin, these preparations dry to form a flexible film. They provide a vehicle for the active ingredients while also acting as a protective dressing. A salicylic acid collodion, for example, is used for the removal of warts.

Topical antifungal treatments

These are used to treat fungal infections such as athlete's foot and candidal diaper rash (thrush), and work by damaging the fungal cell walls, causing them to die. Creams should be applied two to four times daily, as directed. To prevent relapse, these treatments should be continued for one to four weeks after lesions have healed. See individual packs for recommended times.

COMMON **MEDICATIONS...**

Athlete's foot
Lamisil (active ingredient, terbinafine)
Tinactin (active ingredient, tolnaftate)
Lotrimin, Mycelex (active ingredient, clotrimazole)
Monistat, Micatin (active ingredient, miconazole)
Nizoral (active ingredient, ketoconazole)

Candidal diaper rash
Mycostatin (active ingredient, nystatin)

FOR FUNGAL INFECTIONS

EMOLLIENTS

In the United States, emollients made to an official standard formulation will have the letters USP after them (United States Pharmacopoeia). These products, which are cheap to buy, can be as effective as more expensive proprietary preparations. Some of the more commonly used emollients, available both over the counter and by prescription, include:

Standard formulations

Hydrophilic ointment USP An oil in water emulsion. Can be used as an emollient or as a vehicle for other ingredients.

Cold cream USP An oil in water emulsion. Can be used as an emollient or as a vehicle for other ingredients.

White petrolatum USP (white petroleum jelly)

Yellow petrolatum USP (yellow petroleum jelly, Vaseline)

Zinc oxide ointment USP; Calamine lotion USP These both contain zinc oxide, which has mild astringent, soothing and protective effects.

Proprietary emollients

Alpha Keri bath emollient Contains liquid petrolatum and lanolin.

Aveeno cream and bath emollient Contains oatmeal.

Cutemol cream Contains liquid petrolatum, lanolin and beeswax.

Lacticare lotion Contains lactic acid.

Oilatum cleansing bar and soap-free lotion The cleansing bar contains arachis oil (peanut oil). The soap-free cleansing lotion contains antibacterial ingredients for use with infected eczema.

Topical emollients

These mixtures of water, fats, vegetable or mineral oils, and waxes are used to soothe, soften and moisturize the skin. Because of this, they are the first line of treatment for itchy or dry skin conditions such as eczema. They are often used as a base for other skin preparations.

Emollients work by forming a protective film on the surface of your child's skin, which traps water within the skin and keeps it hydrated. They also have a soothing, anti-itching and anti-inflammatory action. Emollients are available as creams, ointments, lotions and soap substitutes, and many different formulations are available both over the counter and by prescription. Several preparations may need to be tried before a suitable one is found for your child's skin.

Because their effects are short lived, emollients should be applied little and often throughout the day. The best time to apply them is after your child has a bath or shower, when the skin is still moist, and then everytime you feed or change your child. Emollients should be applied to the skin in smooth downward strokes in the direction of hair growth. When using an emollient or soap substitute in the bath or shower, gently massage it into your child's skin then rinse it off with clean, warm water to remove any dead skin or crusts.

Emollients may have other ingredients added, such as urea, which hydrates the skin. In some cases, these ingredients may be irritating or cause an allergic reaction.

THE FINGERTIP METHOD FOR STEROID APPLICATION

This useful method for estimating how much topical corticosteroid to use on your child's skin is based on the "fingertip dosing unit" — one unit being equal to about $1/2$ g of steroid. This amount is easy to calculate, as it is the amount of cream that covers an adult finger from the tip to the first crease. The number of units needed to cover different areas of a 4-year-old child are shown opposite. Older children will need slightly more, and younger children slightly less — always read the label to find the exact amount.

Area of the body	Units	Grams
● Face and neck	1	$1/2$ g
● One arm	1	$1/2$ g
● Trunk (front and back)	4	2 g
● Both hands and feet	1	$1/2$ g
● One leg	2	1 g

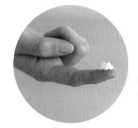

One fingertip unit (about $1/2$ g)

Topical corticosteroids

These are related to hormones produced in the adrenal glands, and like the naturally produced hormones, topical corticosteroids prevent the release of chemicals that trigger inflammation, allowing blood vessels to return to normal, and reducing any swelling. They are used for treating inflammatory conditions, particularly eczema.

Corticosteroid safety

Parents sometimes get anxious about using topical steroids on their children. However, you should not confuse them with anabolic steroids, which are sometimes taken as "body builders," or with oral steroids. Corticosteroids do have side effects — some can thin the skin if used for long periods, and strong topical steroids may also have internal effects if used over a long period. But if applied correctly, they can be invaluable in reducing inflammation and speeding healing in conditions such as eczema. The use of topical steroids for psoriasis is more controversial, since the symptoms return when the medication is stopped, encouraging long-term use.

Application

Always apply an emollient to your child's skin at least half an hour before using the steroid, in order to soften the skin. Then, wearing disposable gloves, smear a thin amount of steroid over the affected areas. Use the fingertip method to measure the quantity (see box, above). Apply the steroid once or twice daily.

COMMON **MEDICATIONS** ...

Generally, these are the lowest strength necessary to achieve a cure. Very potent steroids are rarely used for children.

Mild Hydrocortisone 1 percent (can be used on your child's face)

Moderate Desonide

Potent Betamethasone

Very potent Clobetasol

CORTICOSTEROIDS

surgical treatments

Although most skin problems either disappear on their own or with medications, surgery may be beneficial, or even essential, for some conditions. It's common to be apprehensive about your child having surgical treatment, but in most cases, surgery is minor and done on an outpatient basis under a local anesthetic. This may be by injection or by applying an anesthetic cream to the skin area. With very small children, a general anesthetic would be used, if necessary. Before agreeing to any surgical treatment, make sure you discuss with your doctor the pain involved, the end results and the possibility of side effects such as scarring.

Going into the hospital

If your child does need in-patient treatment, his or her age, personality and any previous hospital experience will affect how he or she reacts to the experience. Younger children may find it difficult to understand why they cannot go home, and many children, particularly if they have never been to the hospital before, may feel anxious and disorientated. You need to explain what's going to happen at your child's particular level of understanding. Most hospitals encourage parents

HANDY **HINTS** ...

The unfamiliar setting of a hospital can seem strange or overwhelming to a young child. Get your child used to the idea of going to the hospital by playing doctors and nurses with a toy medical kit. Reading books with hospital stories, appropriate to your child's level of understanding, can also help make a stay seem less frightening.

PREPARING YOUR CHILD

Prepare for a trip to the hospital by getting your child to bandage a doll or listen for teddy's "heartbeat."

to stay overnight with young children, but if you are not able to be with your child all the time, you should make sure the staff know your child's word for the toilet, any food or drink that he or she dislikes or anything else you think is important. Before your child is discharged, make sure you understand how to do any home treatments that may need to be carried out, such as changing dressings, and any special precautions that are necessary.

Cauterization

This is the deliberate destruction of tissue by careful, local application of heat. It may be used for persistent warts in conjunction with curettage (see right), or for small facial warts using a fine needle as an alternative to cryotherapy (see below). Cauterization is the treatment of choice for the long, threadlike filiform warts, often found on the face, though it may sometimes cause scarring.

Cryotherapy

The destruction of tissue by freezing is known as cryotherapy or cryosurgery. It is mainly used for warts and verrucae, and for molluscum contagiosum. The two main agents used are liquid nitrogen and carbon dioxide snow (dry ice), which are applied either with a cotton-tipped stick, or with a spray. Carbon dioxide has now been mainly superseded by liquid nitrogen. Freezing does not kill wart viruses; it destroys the tissue the virus lives in, so multiple treatments may be necessary.

Cryotherapy treatment is painful and may result in blisters, scarring or hypopigmentation (loss of color from the skin). Children under 10 years of age do not tolerate treatment well and many dermatologists believe cryotherapy is not justified for children.

Curettage

This involves scraping or spooning out foreign matter from a cavity using a spoon-shaped instrument known as a curette. Curettage may be used for skin problems such as molluscum contagiosum, where the soft center is removed from the bumps. It may also be done for persistent or painful warts in conjunction with cautery. An anesthetic cream is applied first, but the procedure may be painful and leave scarring.

Excision

Here a skin lesion is cut off and completely removed. This could include removing a growth such as a mole or hemangioma if it causes problems. Excision may also be done for cosmetic reasons if a growth is in a place where it is causing your child embarrassment, or if other treatments have failed. The removal of a sample of tissue for microscopic analysis to confirm a diagnosis is called a skin biopsy.

Laser surgery

Lasers can be used to cut skin lesions, coagulate or rupture blood vessels and vaporize or otherwise destroy tissue with great accuracy. In particular, laser treatment has revolutionized the management of birthmarks such as port-wine stains and hemangiomas. Laser light is different from ordinary light: A conventional lightbulb emits light of varying wavelengths in all directions, but all the light waves in lasers are of the same wavelength, so it spreads out very little and is intensely concentrated. This intensity may be increased further by the use of a focusing mechanism to target a small area of skin.

There are many different types of lasers, using different materials to produce and amplify the light: dye lasers produce light by energizing a liquid colored with dye; neodymium YAG lasers use crystal; other lasers uses gases such as argon

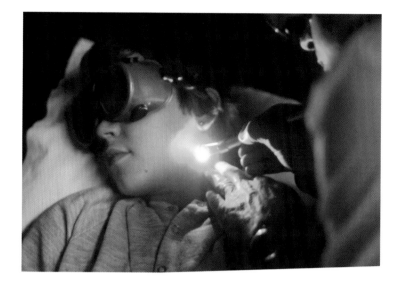

New advances in laser surgery have made the treatment safer, more sensitive and more effective, and it is now used to treat an increasing number of childhood skin conditions.

or carbon dioxide. The type used will depend on the problem and on the need to avoid unwanted effects on skin pigmentation. The light from carbon dioxide lasers, for example, is absorbed by water in body tissue, while dye and argon lasers produce light that is absorbed by pigmented tissue, making them useful for treating birthmarks. Dye lasers are particularly suitable for children, because there is less risk of scarring than with other lasers.

Dye lasers

Surface stains on the skin such as port-wine stains and pigmented lesions can be removed with dye lasers. The dye is altered, depending on the skin pigment targeted, to produce light that is absorbed by tissue. Pigments in the tissue absorb the wavelengths of laser light and produce heat. This causes damage to the pigmented cells or blood vessels. The brown pigment melanin may be targeted if there is a birthmark such as a brown patch, or the red blood pigment if the mark is a port-wine stain. Pulsed-dye lasers, which deliver light in very short bursts, are most commonly used for port-wine stains. Over a period of months, the damaged vessels are replaced by colorless tissue, resulting in a decrease in blood flow and a subsequent paling of your child's birthmark.

Treatment may begin as soon as your child is old enough for day-case general anesthesia. Ideally this should start between 6 and 12 months. About 80 percent of children with port-wine stains will respond well to laser treatment, but results are variable and there may not be complete clearance of the stain. Multiple treatments may be needed and advice on aftercare should be followed carefully.

Side effects of laser treatments

During the treatment there may be some stinging or pain, and this may be followed after treatment by a burning sensation or sometimes swelling. After pulsed-dye treatment, a blue-gray discoloration resembling a bruise may occur, although some newer lasers use a slightly longer wavelength to minimize or prevent bruising. Possible complications of laser treatment include alterations of the skin pigment and scarring.

complementary therapies

An increasingly popular option in the treatment of skin problems, complementary therapies can often be used together with, or even in place of, conventional ones. Popular herbal remedies such as witch hazel or calendula cream have been used for many years and are considered gentle and safe for children. However, concern has been expressed that some preparations used in complementary therapies are not licensed, unlike "conventional" medicinal substances.

Herbalism

Humans have been using plants for medicinal purposes since the dawn of time, and herbal medicine, or phytotherapy as it is sometimes known, is one of the oldest forms of medicine. If you want to use a herbal medicine to treat your child's skin problem, always consult a qualified

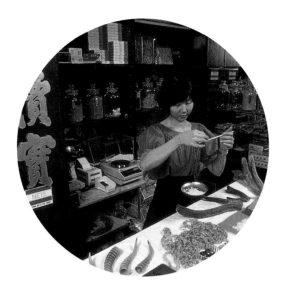

Many traditional Chinese medicines are very effective, but they are not always well regulated.

herbalist and inform your doctor — although herbal preparations are "natural," not all of them are safe. Some internal preparations can be dangerous or react with conventional medicines. Some plants can also cause a skin reaction.

Chinese medicine

In recent years there has been a surge of interest in the use of traditional Chinese medicine (TCM) for the treatment of skin complaints, particularly eczema, and there is no doubt that for some people these preparations are useful. However, concerns have been expressed about the toxicity of some of these medicines, and the fact that these preparations are not licensed. Recent research published in the *British Medical Journal* suggests many herbal creams contain a high concentration of a topical steroid inappropriate for children. Dermatologists recommend that Chinese medicine should be used only under strict medical supervision and is best restricted to those with severe eczema that is unresponsive to conventional treatment.

HEALTH CHECK ...

Always consult a registered practitioner before beginning a course of complementary therapy, and do not stop using conventional preparations such as emollients or steroids without your doctor's approval. Always check the ingredients of preparations before use, and test the preparation on a small area of clear skin 24 hours before applying it properly. If the skin reacts, do not use. Stop using any preparation that seems to make your child's condition worse.

COMPLEMENTARY THERAPY

DIET

In some cases, what your child eats may play a part in his or her skin condition. If you suspect important foods such as wheat or dairy products are making your child's skin problem worse, you may wish to talk to your doctor about cutting them out. Don't be tempted to put your child on an exclusion diet without consulting your doctor: a restricted diet could lead to other health problems. Excluding minor foods such as oranges or tomatoes, or drinks such as cola from your child's diet will not, however, cause health problems.

Homeopathy

Based upon the use of minute doses of substances to boost the body's defenses, homeopathy uses the theory of treating "like with like" — the idea that a complaint can be treated with a substance that would produce symptoms of that illness in a healthy person. Most preparations are made to be taken orally, but external applications are available for a number of skin problems and are available from pharmacies and health shops.

Homeopathic remedies are safe, but should not be used in place of conventional medicines for serious skin conditions or infectious rashes. If you want to treat your child's skin problem with an internal remedy, always inform your doctor and consult a qualified homeopathic doctor.

USEFUL HERBAL REMEDIES

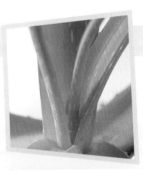

Many herbal and homeopathic creams and lotions, useful for minor skin complaints, are available over the counter.

◀ **ALOE VERA LOTION** helps soothes inflamed skin and insect bites.

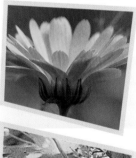

ARNICA is effective for bruises. Do not use on broken skin.

◀ **CALENDULA** is antiseptic and antifungal and can be used for diaper rash, minor cuts and grazes, minor burns and itchy skin.

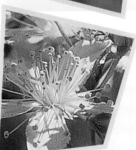

◀ **HYPERICUM** (Saint-John's-wort) is soothing and anti-inflammatory, and can be applied to bruises, bites and stings.

WITCH HAZEL LOTION is soothing and mildly astringent. It can be used as a compress or dabbed on bruises, bites, stings and cold sores.

Aromatherapy

Essential oils are aromatic essences extracted from a wide variety of herbs, flowers and trees. They have been shown to be effective in the treatment of certain skin problems such as eczema and fungal infections, and often make a useful alternative or addition to orthodox treatments. The essences are very concentrated, and most need to be mixed with a base oil such as sweet almond. Many base oils have useful emollient properties — jojoba, which is a wax, is particularly good for eczema.

Always buy good quality oils, and store them in dark glass bottles, in a cool, dark place. When used correctly, most oils are safe, but a few have risks. Some are known to be toxic, some may cause irritation and some are unsuitable for young children. Consult a trained aromatherapist before using oils if your child has a serious health problem, allergies or sensitive skin, or if you are pregnant. Essential oils must never be taken internally, so keep them locked up and well out of reach of curious children. Also, make sure you do not use oils or blends on or near broken skin.

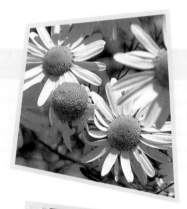

USEFUL ESSENTIAL OILS

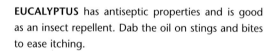

◄ **CAMOMILE** is calming and soothing. It is useful for skin problems such as insect bites and minor burns and for soothing cold sores.

EUCALYPTUS has antiseptic properties and is good as an insect repellent. Dab the oil on stings and bites to ease itching.

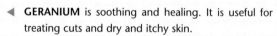

◄ **GERANIUM** is soothing and healing. It is useful for treating cuts and dry and itchy skin.

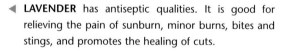

◄ **LAVENDER** has antiseptic qualities. It is good for relieving the pain of sunburn, minor burns, bites and stings, and promotes the healing of cuts.

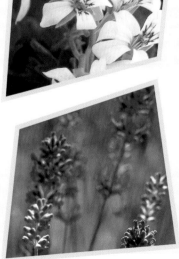

TEA TREE is a nonirritating antiseptic said to kill bacteria, fungi and viruses. Dab on spots and pimples, boils, cold sores, cuts and abrasions, and athlete's foot.

How to treat your child

Oils can be blended and massaged into the skin or applied in a compress or lotion, but apart from lavender for minor cuts and burns and tea tree for spots, cold sores and fungal infections, undiluted oils must never be applied directly to the skin. Oils can also be added to a bath or foot bath, or inhaled from a bowl of hot water. Make sure your child keeps his or her eyes closed, as injury can result if oil vapors get in the eyes.

MAKING A COMPRESS

1 Add four to eight drops of essential oil to 1 pint (500 ml) of hand-hot water in a bowl. Stir the water until the oil disperses evenly.

2 Take a piece of absorbent cloth, such as muslin, and lay it on the surface of the water so that it can soak up the liquid.

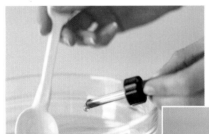
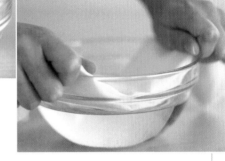

3 Place the compress over the affected area and cover with towels. It's best to do this when your child is happy to stay calm and still for 10 to 15 minutes.

MAKING A BLEND

2 Pour the blended oils into your hands and massage into the affected areas of your child's skin using small circular strokes.

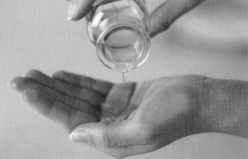

1 Take 3 tablespoons (45 ml) of a base or carrier oil, such as almond, jojoba, wheat germ or peach kernel oil. Add 3 drops of the recommended essential oil.

home remedies

It is not always necessary to treat your child with expensive, commercially formulated products. Many childhood skin problems can be soothed or relieved using ingredients that may be found in any kitchen cabinet, meaning you can treat your child's ailment promptly without having to leave the house. Although these remedies should never be used as a substitute for proper medical attention, for minor problems they are often as effective as anything found in a pharmacy.

HONEY can help draw pus out of infected wounds and bring boils to a head.

CUCUMBER slices can be used as a poultice for cooling sunburn and minor insect stings.

BAKING SODA (Bicarbonate of soda) helps relieve itching, and is useful for bites and nettle rash. Mix enough water to make a paste that will cling to the skin, and leave on for 15 to 20 minutes.

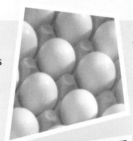

EGGS can help to relieve minor sunburn or a sore diaper rash. Apply the egg whites to the skin in layers, allowing each layer to dry.

EPSOM SALTS can help relieve itching from insect bites. Dissolve 1 tablespoon (15 ml) in one quart (1 L) of hot water and then cool. Dip a cloth into the solution and place on the bite for 15 to 20 minutes.

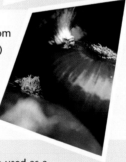

ONIONS, used crushed or sliced, help soothe wasp stings. To clear warts, dab twice daily with the onion juice.

CABBAGE LEAVES can be used as a poultice to relieve boils, blisters and stings. Discard the ribs and crush fresh leaves with a rolling pin. Secure to the skin with a bandage.

GARLIC makes an excellent antifungal agent, and can be applied, either as juice or in a clove, to mild athlete's foot. Also useful for warts.

VINEGAR is useful for soothing the skin and relieving the pain of minor sunburn. Also can be dabbed on wasp stings.

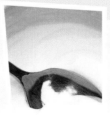

YOGURT (natural) soothes the skin and can help relieve the pain of minor sunburn. Add a couple of drops of lavender oil for greater effect.

It isn't always convenient to leave your home, especially if your child is ill. But there are natural, soothing remedies to be found in most homes.

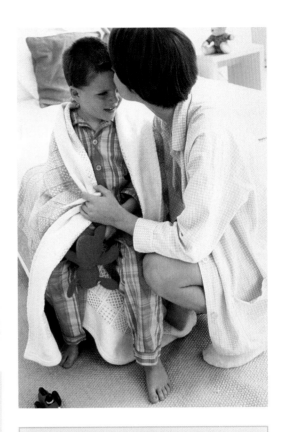

LEMON JUICE offers useful relief from warts, cold sores and wasp stings.

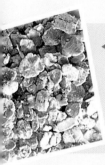

◀ **OATMEAL** helps to soothe itchy skin caused by conditions such as eczema or chickenpox. Add a handful to your child's bath water.

BREAD can be used to bring boils to a head and remove crusting. Cut into small pieces, put into a pan with a little milk or water, and simmer for a few minutes. Wring out in a cotton cloth until all excess liquid is removed, and apply to the skin.

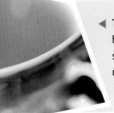

◀ **TEA**, applied black and cold, can help heal cold sores. Dab on the sores or use a wet tea bag as a ready-made compress.

LEEKS can help to relieve the soreness of insect stings. Rub a slice into your child's skin at the site of the sting.

MAKING A POULTICE

These are similar to compresses (see p.87), but are made as a soft paste with the surplus liquid wrung out, and have a more drawing effect.

The paste is usually applied hot, between a piece of cloth or gauze, or applied directly onto the affected part. Hold the poultice in place by hand, or secure it with some type of wrapping, such as a bandage.

CREAMS

You can make your own soothing creams by mixing a little of a suitable herbal tincture, decoction or infusion, or a few drops of essential oil, into a base cream such as aqueous or emulsifying cream.

potential irritants

There are a huge number of potentially irritating substances, which may cause your child problems such as itching, eczema or dermatitis. Identifying these is often a matter of trial and error, particularly as your child may use a product or eat a certain food for a long time before developing a reaction to it. Some children may even be allergic to a substance in a product designed to help cure skin problems, such as the lanolin used in some moisturizers. Itchy or inflamed skin can also result from the action of physical stimuli such as pressure or friction, or factors such as cold, heat or stress.

If you suspect a product is causing your child irritation, try not using it for a few days to see if the problem improves. You should never omit an important food such as milk or wheat from a child's diet for more than a few days without first checking with a doctor.

This chart gives examples of some of the substances most commonly implicated in childhood skin rashes and irritation.

HOUSE DUST MITES
This common indoor irritant can be found in mattresses, furniture and carpets. Frequent vacuuming and use of a mattress cover may be necessary.

PETS
Cat or dog hair or other animal furs, or even contact with animal saliva, may cause your child problems.

RUBBER
Chemicals in some types of rubber, sometimes found in watch straps, may irritate your child's skin.

METALS
A rash around your child's neck, wrist, waist or ears may indicate a reaction to metals such as nickel, copper, chromium or cobalt, since these are often used in jewelry, in belt buckles or for the studs on jeans.

FOOD AND DRINK
Common culprits include milk, soya, strawberries, shellfish and other seafood, peanuts, spices, chocolate, tea, eggs and food additives.

◄ CHEMICALS IN CREAMS AND MOISTURIZERS

Many skin care products and cosmetics contain chemicals and other substances that can cause irritation, such as benzyl benzoate, lanolin, beeswax and many fragrances.

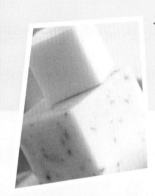

◄ SOAPS AND DETERGENTS

Even soaps that contain no fragrances or additives may strip your child's skin of oils. If your child's skin is very dry, try using a soap-free emollient instead. Use gentle detergents and make sure your child's clothes are properly rinsed after washing.

PLANTS

Poison ivy, nettles, grass pollens, tree pollens and mold spores are all common causes of childhood skin rashes. Some garden plants and flowers, such as chrysanthemums and geraniums, may also irritate your child's skin.

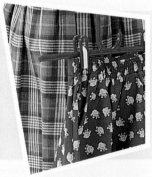

◄ CLOTHING

Coarse fabrics such as wool can easily irritate your child's sensitive skin. You should also avoid dressing your child in tight-fitting clothing, especially if made with synthetic materials. If freshly laundered clothing seems to be causing irritation, the problem may be with the detergent, and the clothes will need to be well rinsed.

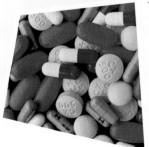

◄ DRUGS

Almost any medication, whether rubbed into the skin or taken orally, can potentially cause a reaction. Penicillin hypersensitivity is very common, but aspirin, other antibiotics, codeine, nonsteroidal anti-inflammatories and local anesthetics also often cause a reaction.

glossary

Acute An illness or condition with a rapid, sudden or severe onset. The opposite of chronic.

Allergen Any substance that causes an allergic reaction.

Allergy An inappropriate or abnormal reaction by the body's immune system to a substance, such as a food, plant or medication, that is normally harmless.

Analgesic A medicine used to prevent or treat pain. These may range from mild and safe drugs such as acetaminophen, to powerful and sometimes dangerous drugs such as morphine. Although aspirin is a mild analgesic, it should not be given to children under 16, unless prescribed by a doctor.

Antibiotic A drug used to treat infections caused by bacteria. It is important to complete a prescribed course, o prevent bacteria developing immunity. Antibiotics do not work for viral infections.

Antibodies Also known as immunoglobulin (Ig) antibodies. Small, Y-shaped structures produced by the immune system to fight infections.

Antihistamine A drug used to relieve symptoms of an allergic reaction such as urticaria, or to relieve itching. It works by blocking the action of histamine, a chemical released by the body during an allergic reaction.

Astringent A substance or drug that shrinks and tightens the skin cells.

Atopy A predisposition or hereditary tendency to allergies such as asthma, hay fever or eczema.

Bacteria A microorganism that lives in the environment. There are thousands of different types of bacteria: some may cause an infection or disease, such as meningitis or impetigo, while others are harmless or "friendly."

Benign Not cancerous or malignant.

Biopsy The process of taking a specimen of tissue from the body, for examination under a microscope.

Candida Commonly called thrush, candida is an infection caused by the fungus *Candida albicans*, a yeast fungus that can cause a type of diaper rash in babies.

Chronic The opposite of acute. A chronic illness is one of long duration.

Collagen A fibrous protein that gives the skin its firmness.

Complication A disease or problem that arises from the original illness. For example, meningitis may occur as a result of measles.

Congenital A condition that is present at birth.

Contagious Used to describe a disease that can be caught from another person — an infectious disease.

Dermatitis Inflamed skin that may be caused by contact with an irritant or allergen.

Dermis The thicker and deeper, inner layer of the skin, which is mainly composed of collagen.

Epidermis The thin, upper, outer layer of the skin, made up of several layers of cells.

Fungi Complex organisms capable, in some cases, of causing skin diseases such as ringworm, athlete's foot or candida (thrush).

Hormones Chemicals produced by various glands or organs in the body and released into the bloodstream to another part of the body, where they exert some kind of effect. During puberty, for example, the level of hormones called androgens rises, stimulating the sebaceous glands and causing an overproduction of sebum, which may lead in turn to blocked ducts and acne.

Immunization The process, either natural or artificial, whereby people become immune to specific infectious diseases. Natural immunity occurs when an individual catches an infectious disease and produces antibodies against the microorganisms causing the infection. Artificial immunity occurs when an individual is made immune to a disease by vaccination, without actually experiencing the full disease.

Immunoglobulin See *Antibodies.*

Incubation The period between exposure to an infection and the appearance of the first symptoms.

Infectious A disease that can spread and be caught by someone else. See *Contagious.*

Malignant A cancerous growth, such as a melanoma.

Melanin A pigment that gives the skin its color, and helps protect against ultraviolet rays.

Nevus A type of birthmark resulting in a skin discoloration or swelling on any part of the body. They may be present at birth, such as a port-wine stain; appear shortly after birth, such as a strawberry mark; or be acquired as the child grows older, such as freckles.

Sebaceous glands These produce an oily substance called sebum, which lubricates the hair and forms a protective film over the skin, preventing it from drying out.

Sebum Oil produced by the sebaceous glands to keep the hair and skin lubricated.

Topical For application directly onto the skin. For example, corticosteroid or antihistamine cream may be used to treat a child's rash topically, as opposed to taking steroid or antihistamine tablets by mouth (orally).

Vaccine A preparation containing infectious organisms that have been modified or killed, so that they stimulate the immune system into producing antibodies to protect the body against a certain disease, without actually causing the disease itself.

Vascular Pertaining to blood or blood vessels.

Virus A tiny, infectious organism, which can reproduce only by invading a living cell.

Yeast Single-celled plants which are classified as fungi and which can cause skin infections such as candida.

index

acknowledgments

I would like to express my thanks to everyone who has helped with the production of this book. In particular, thanks to editor Tom Broder for his help, encouragement and unfailing good humor.

I would also like to thank all the mothers I have met as a health visitor over the years, whose many and varied questions on their children's skin problems first raised my interest in this topic and gave me an idea of the need for such a book. I hope they will find it useful.

June Thompson

The publishers would like to thank:
Production Karol Davies and Nigel Reed
Computer Support Paul Stradling
Picture Research Sandra Schneider
Photography Jules Selmes

picture credits

1 (bottom left) medipics; 9 Francoise Sauze/SPL; 12 (left) Mark Clarke/SPL; (right) BSIP Laurent/SPL; 14 Saturn Stills/SPL; 15 Dr I Williams; 16 (right) Wellcome Trust Photographic Library; 17 Chris Priest/SPL; 18 (bottom) Creatas; 20 Dr I Williams; 22 Damien Lovegrove/SPL; 23 James King-Holmes/SPL; 24 (left) Dr I Williams; (right) Dr P Marazzi/SPL; 27 Dr I Williams; 29 Bubbles/Ian West; 30 Dr I Williams; 31 CNRI/SPL; 32 (left) John Radcliffe Hospital/SPL (right) Mike Peres/Custom Medical Stock Photo/SPL; 33 (left) Dr I Williams (right) Dr P Marazzi/SPL; 34 Dr I Williams; 35 Dr I Williams; 38 (left) Dr I Williams (right) Custom Medical Stock Photo/SPL; 39 Dr I Williams; 40 Dr I Williams; 41 Dr I Williams; 42 Wellcome Trust Medical Photographic Library; 43 Meningitis Trust; 44 Lowell Georgia/SPL; 45 Dr I Williams; 46 Dr I Williams; 47 Jules Selmes; 48 (left) Dr I Williams (right) Biophoto Associates/SPL; 49 Dr I Williams; 50 Dr I Williams; 51 St Bartholomew's Hospital/SPL; 52 Dr I Williams; 53 (left) Dr Jeremy Burgess/SPL; (right) Mark Clarke/SPL; 54 Hattie Young/SPL; 56 Dr Jeremy Burgess/SPL; 57 Dr I Williams; 58 Dr P Marazzi/SPL; 60 Dr Chris Hale/SPL; 61 Dr I Williams; 62 (top) John Eastcott and Yva Momatiuk/SPL; (bottom) Andrew Syred/SPL; 64 (top) Dr P Marazzi/SPL; (bottom) medipics; 65 Dr P Marazzi/SPL; 66 SPL; 68 (top) Dr P Marazzi/SPL; (bottom) Biophoto Associates/SPL; 70 medipics; 71 Dr I Williams; 72 Dr I Williams; 73 Dr P Marazzi/SPL; 74 Dr I Williams; 76 Chris Priest/SPL; 81 Powerstock; 83 Dr Rob Stepney/Aumer/SPL; 84 Will and Deni McIntyre/SPL; 89 (top right) Getty Images; 90 (centre) CNRI/SPL; **Front jacket** Jules Selmes